Health Colonialism

Forerunners: Ideas First

Short books of thought-in-process scholarship, where intense analysis, questioning, and speculation take the lead

FROM THE UNIVERSITY OF MINNESOTA PRESS

(Continued on page 100)

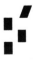

Health Colonialism
Urban Wastelands and
Hospital Frontiers

Shiloh Krupar

University of Minnesota Press
MINNEAPOLIS
LONDON

ISBN 978-1-5179-1542-1 (pb)
ISBN 978-1-4529-6961-9 (Ebook)
ISBN 978-1-4529-6962-6 (Manifold)

Published by the University of Minnesota Press, 2023
111 Third Avenue South, Suite 290
Minneapolis, MN 55401-2520
www.upress.umn.edu

Available as a Manifold edition at manifold.umn.edu

Contents

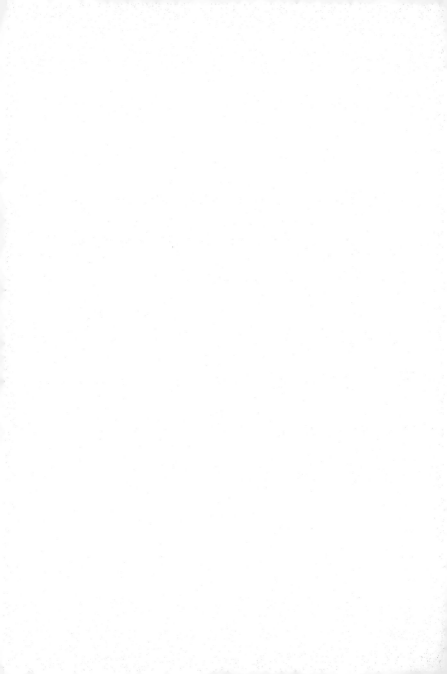

Introduction

THE UNEVEN DEVASTATION of the Covid-19 pandemic shows how different life conditions shape health. From Covid data dashboards to virtual and physical memorials honoring the deceased, efforts to reckon with the pandemic—algorithmic and embodied alike—evince the disparate impacts of the disease. The phrase "social determinants of health" attempts to convey, soberly and irrefutably, that the environments and relationships wherein people are born and live affect health risks and outcomes.[1] Vast inequalities among populations lead to different coronavirus susceptibility and survival rates. Within the health arena, scholars, practitioners, and policy makers advocate the framework of "structural violence" to heed the power relations that undergird such grossly divergent life chances. Simultaneous with the pandemic sweeping across the globe in 2020, calls to "decolonize health" repeatedly surfaced in hashtags, academic articles, and health organization public statements.[2] Importantly, these critiques acknowledge the central role

1. U.S. Department of Health and Human Services, "Social Determinants of Health," accessed November 7, 2022, https://health.gov/healthypeople/priority-areas/social-determinants-health.
2. Mishal Khan, Seye Abimbola, Tammam Aloudat, Emanuele Capobianco, Sarah Hawkes, and Afifah Rahman-Shepherd, "Decolonising Global Health in 2021: A Roadmap to Move from Rhetoric to Reform," *BMJ Global Health* 6, no. 3 (2021): 1.

that medicine and medical institutions have historically played in colonialism: tropical medicine to protect colonizers and cordon sanitaires to secure borders; epidemiology and inoculations that buffer industry, trade, and military activity. The analytic scope, however, remains limited to institutional politics and the unbalanced partnerships between Global North and Global South. A biomedical framework that partitions medicine and technology from ecology, culture, politics, and economy dominates solutions and champions social responsibility. This obscures the ways that contemporary medicine advances colonial relations of health disparity.[3]

In response to these efforts and the pandemic, this volume foregrounds health colonialism. I position U.S. biomedicine as a colonial frontier and U.S. hospitals as settler-colonial institutions driven by extractive racial-capitalist logics that dominate space with health effects. I look at the political geographies of social determinants of health, specifically how property relations organize waste and race and entrench settler and anti-Black domination. I thus consider health colonialism in terms of land as property and as pedagogy (as blight, public use, etc.), and in doing so denaturalize liberal assumptions about health and the structural violence of U.S. health care. The arc of the analysis shows how land policies and development practices of American hospitals succeed in concentrating capital via parasitical relations with place locally and with other national health systems transnationally by providing expensive acute and emergency care within the United States' minimal social safety net. This entrenches a global color line connecting domestic land grabs to elite medical hubs as interrelated forms of health colonialism. In other words, domestic health colonialism of ur-

3. I use "biomedicine" and "medicine" interchangeably in this text, but biomedicalization temporally marks the shift in medicine toward privatization and corporatization, increasingly technoscientific practices, and intensification of health/biomedical knowledges across social domains. See Adele E. Clarke, Laura Mamo, Jennifer Ruth Fosket, Jennifer R. Fishman, and Janet K. Shim, eds., *Biomedicalization: Technoscience, Health, and Illness in the U.S.* (Durham, N.C.: Duke University Press, 2010).

ban centers serves as the material-extractive basis for globalizing U.S. biomedicine and health trade. It supports medical entrepôts that further divide the medical haves from the have-nots while claiming that the benefits of globalizing health services and trade will trickle down. Any challenges to mounting medical apartheid globally must question social relations of land/property and health as well as the globalization of U.S. biomedicine.

There is a dearth of attention to the land practices and territorial operations of U.S. hospitals. This is surprising, given that top-tier hospitals have been expanding their clinical practices in the form of massive inner-city health campuses and overseas hospital franchises. These development projects use enormous resources, land, and labor; receive tax breaks and other incentives in the name of charity and philanthropy; and seek to generate wealth and trade on brand-name expertise through domestic operations that rely on local assets. This volume attends to this lacuna by examining land redevelopment projects led by U.S. hospitals. The book surveys the real estate practices of hospitals and queries their role in gentrification and land revitalization, the massive public subsidies and infrastructure they require, and the ways that elite nonprofit U.S. hospitals have carved out real estate empires in their host cities to underwrite international prospecting for patients, transnational specialty clinics, and overseas hospitality services. The account scrutinizes how elite hospitals actively perpetuate conditions of poverty and ill health in their surrounding neighborhoods even as their philanthropic/civilizing missions and nonprofit status rhetorically obscure harmful effects, be they industrial pollution or escalating local disease and morbidity rates. In this way, hospital land redevelopment projects may profit from the very blight that they claim to remedy.

I examine policies that seek to build hospitals on contaminated land and, more generally, that facilitate land seizures in the name of improving public use and environmental health. These policies propagate a colonial process that identifies certain spaces as blighted—a racially charged discourse in the United States that has resulted in repeated struggles over so-called public use and civic benefits. Using a critical geographical framework that addresses racial capitalism and settler colonialism, the account focuses on the racially inequitable political-economic operations of these medical institutions and their effects on neighborhood spaces and livelihoods. The analysis registers the damages of land dispossession in order to establish property and pollution as central to health colonialism, and to show the material and pedagogical ties between waste, land, and race made by health institutions that pursue urban expansion projects. I specifically scrutinize how particular medical centers and hospitals create a frontier of contaminated or underutilized land parcels primed for redevelopment via financial incentives that limit liability in the private property market and strip assets from communities, all while averring public improvements. Drawing on the policy term "brownfields," I call this frontier "medical brownfields" (see chapter 1); I track its consolidation and anchoring of hospitals as transnational investment frontiers within the political economy of U.S. empire and biomedicine.

Globalization has challenged the national "containerization" of health systems. The book plumbs hospital policy literature and political-economic practices that inaugurate global medical hubs—from Las Vegas to Abu Dhabi—and that function as international economic and educational ventures. These satellite hospitals trade medical expertise, procedures, supply chains, financial practices, and land strategies while in the process tethering the prestige of these elite hospitals and their international outposts to the reproduction of domestic blight and inequality across borders. This transnational extension of medical brownfields stratifies territory and populations, consolidating the locally extractive, environmentally damaging work of this frontier to buoy branded medical services and the so-called global medical commons. Thus, campaigns to decolonize health must address hospital land practices and the territorial, socioenvironmental effects of their medical services and clinical practices across scales of operation.

In what follows, I discuss three policy fields that support hospital development projects. Chapter 1 establishes the settler-colonial and racial-capitalist nature of medical real estate projects by focusing on brownfield property revitalization and the relationships between waste, race, and health. The analysis extends to what is known as healthfields policy that offers hospitals tax breaks and other incentives to redevelop contaminated land in neighborhoods with limited medical services. The policy aims to enhance public health yet in practice can target minority communities and lower liability to remedy toxic blight, thus ensuring that possible contamination continues to endanger human health.

Chapter 2 shifts policy terrain to "Eds and Meds" projects that seek to remedy postindustrial blight and that stimulate urban growth tied to medical research centers and teaching hospitals, which are perceived as powerful economic engines. Participating institutions are able to exploit public subsidies and devalued land; they implement predatory forms of financial extraction using the colonial rhetoric of educational mission and nonprofit charity work even as local communities evince some of the worst disease rates in the United States.

Chapter 3 investigates the expansion of U.S. hospital branches and joint ventures that support profit seeking outside the constraints of U.S. charity and emergency care requirements. Particularly where U.S. hospitals open franchises in oil-rich countries and special-service enclaves in the United States that cater to global elites, they compound inequality by extracting domestically to support speculative international projects couched in global cross-cultural exchange and educational mission, thereby intensifying health and environmental inequities.

The conclusion takes up the call to "decolonize health," drawing on Frantz Fanon's anticolonial argument about the centrality of land to health. I point to the inadequacy of Western medicine's ethical imperative to do no harm, which fails to account for the status quo of health colonialism. In a speculative turn that questions what a health system based on "nonkilling"—or, in Fanon's words, "breathing and bread"—would look like, I argue that decolonizing global health requires reckoning with the ways the Western biomedical model stems from the liberal tradition.

1. Urban Brownfields and Health Policy

HEALTH TAKES PLACE WITHIN specific embodied spatial and temporal contexts. It is altered by geographies of power that condition relationships and institutions. It is "an outcome of the physical and social geographies that shape and determine those social determinants [of health] and health care systems."[1] Research and policy increasingly address social determinants of health and the colonial structures of violence that endure in health care access and equity. Yet a lack of attention to the role of land and property means crucial aspects of colonialism remain unknown and thus taken for granted—namely that "enduring colonial structures like private property, land dispossession, and racism . . . define and shape health outcomes immeasurably."[2] Medicine in the United States extends settler colonialism and racial capitalism through the legacies of property and industrial contamination, even as health care aims to ameliorate the embodied harms of those systemic legacies.[3] This chapter seeks

1. Sarah de Leeuw, Sean Maurice, Travis Holyk, Margo Greenwood, and Warner Adam, "With Reserves: Colonial Geographies and First Nations Health," *Annals of the Association of American Geographers* 102, no. 5 (2012): 908.
2. Neil Nunn, "Toxic Encounters, Settler Logics of Elimination, and the Future of a Continent," *Antipode* 50, no. 5 (2018): 1333.
3. I follow Alyosha Goldstein's insight that in "the United States, colonialism and the legacies of racial slavery remain actively constitutive

to denaturalize the land practices that support health care within the political economy of urban redevelopment. Rejecting the biomedical model of health that inoculates medical institutions from the ways they colonize space and expand the frontier operations of urban renewal, I take up the specific policy of brownfield redevelopment to open a conversation about the colonial power relations of property and pollution and their necropolitical operations on Black, Indigenous, and people of color (BIPOC) communities. Brownfields give us insight into the settler-colonial property frontier and its "toxic disregard for life"—that is, racialized processes of spatial production that rely on dehumanization, exclusion/privilege, and acceptance of conditions that expose certain populations to health risks, injury, disease susceptibility, and death.[4] The discussion seeks to foreground land pedagogy and practices, including, first, the moral geographies of improving unproductive (wasteful) land that anchor the settler-colonial state; second, discourses of blight that blame BIPOC communities for their intimate proximity with waste in order to justify land grabs; and third, a vast extension of eminent domain under the auspices of eliminating so-called noxious influences for the public good.[5] Brownfields bring into view the ways that social groups have different capacities to make land into property as a result of regimes of value tied to waste and race.[6] Indeed, this

---

for capitalist accumulation. Colonialism in this context is not or not only a process of expansion and incorporation, but is a primary social, economic, and political feature of the United States itself; a retrospective and prospective feature that works in tandem with U.S. imperial exploits globally." Alyosha Goldstein, "On the Reproduction of Race, Capitalism, and Settler Colonialism," in *Race and Capitalism: Global Territories, Transnational Histories* (Los Angeles: Institute on Inequality and Democracy, University of California, Los Angeles, 2018), 45.

4. Nunn, "Toxic Encounters," 1336, 1342.

5. Wendell E. Pritchett, "The 'Public Menace' of Blight: Urban Renewal and the Private Uses of Eminent Domain," *Yale Law and Policy Review* 21, no. 1 (2003): 26.

6. Sara Safransky, "Rethinking Land Struggle in the Postindustrial City," *Antipode* 49, no. 4 (2017): 1090.

is central to health colonialism, which is actively maintained by existing governmental and political-economic structures, urban land redevelopment, and waste management.

Industrial practices have left widespread contamination affecting land, water, air, and human and nonhuman bodies.[7] Dealing with contaminated land has necessitated mechanisms of land conversion that serve as the foundation for development projects. Land conversions involve complex shifts in meanings, investment structures, policy proposals, institutions, and physical arrangement. It includes legislation aimed at liability for site remediation as well as financial instruments and international agreements that parlay land redevelopment risk between private and public agencies. Over the last few decades, local, state, federal, and transnational policies have promoted the redevelopment of contaminated land using voluntary and market-based policy instruments. Brownfields have emerged as a widespread and prominent mechanism of land conversion in the United States. The term "brownfields" refers to abandoned or underutilized industrial and commercial sites that are, or are perceived to be, physically, chemically, or biologically contaminated. They comprise reused land or property complicated by the (potential) presence of a hazardous substance, pollutant, or contaminant. Such land is often what remains of former industrial and/or military work, but the term is used more broadly to include idle, abandoned, derelict, damaged, vacant, underused land or buildings with poor ground conditions. The term "brownfields" therefore may refer to land with known documented and perceived pollutants and hazardous wastes, or to land that is not being used to the potential of its perceived or imagined value. For advocates, brownfield policies offer not only environmental cleanup but also locally driven land recycling and

7. This chapter draws on Shiloh Krupar, "Brownfields as Waste/ Race Governance: U.S. Contaminated Property Redevelopment and Racial Capitalism," in *The Routledge Handbook of Waste Studies,* edited by Zsuzsa Gille and Josh Lepawsky (London: Routledge, 2022), 238–53.

health improvement, "with the promise to transform distressed sites across the United States from blight to valuable economic and environmental resources."[8]

In the early 1990s, big-city mayors and legislators from urban industrial states pressured Congress and the U.S. Environmental Protection Agency (EPA) to start a pilot program to redevelop underutilized and/or damaged land in highly desirable urban infill areas.[9] These brownfields, which were often cheaper than comparable nonpolluted properties, became sites of promise for reusing a struggling city's vacant or depleted land—as a "green investment" to conserve greenfields (unused land) by redeveloping brownfields. Such properties could become new factories, businesses, housing, and other revenue-creating endeavors. Brownfields may involve more risk, but they offer the prospect of higher rates of return. They usually require special financing as well as risk-transfer mechanisms that enable developers to limit environmental and financial liability. The central premise of most brownfield redevelopment programs is that regulatory flexibility is needed in order to bring contaminated properties back onto the tax rolls—that is, brownfield strategies eschew punitive regulatory models of environmental protection to pursue "cooperative approaches" that encourage voluntary environmental improvements via market-oriented property development.[10] To that end, the EPA first launched a pilot brownfields program in 1995 to support the agency's land revitalization goals of reusing contaminated properties to reinvigorate communities, thus preventing sprawl, preserving green space, and protecting

8. Matthew Dull and Kris Wernstedt, "Land Recycling, Community Revitalization, and Distributive Politics: An Analysis of EPA Brownfields Program Support," *Policy Studies Journal* 38, no. 1 (2010): 120.

9. Michael R. Greenberg and Justin Hollander, "The Environmental Protection Agency's Brownfields Pilot Program," *American Journal of Public Health* 96, no. 2 (2006): 277–81.

10. Kris Wernstedt and Robert Hersh, "'Through a Lens Darkly'— Superfund Spectacles on Public Participation at Brownfield Sites," *Risk* 9, no. 2 (1998): 157; Dull and Wernstedt, "Land Recycling," 136.

the environment.[11] The program was given statutory footing by the 2002 Small Business Liability Relief and Brownfields Revitalization Act. This act provided the EPA pilot with a congressional mandate, clarified liability issues to make redevelopment more attractive, and adopted new tools to promote land conversion; funding was increased to $250 million per year.[12]

In contrast to federal programs that rely predominantly on liability and enforcement to initiate cleanups, brownfield voluntary programs permit site owners and developers to approach the state to identify potentially valuable sites, especially within inner cities. Numerous states have enacted their own brownfields programs, with different mixes of incentives, regulatory pressure, information provision, and public involvement. These programs typically limit cleanup costs and responsibility for adverse consequences of land conversion; they also imply that there will be job creation in economically distressed areas, along with improvements in environmental health. Cities and other planning authorities draw on federal seed funding and state programs to apply advanced appraisal techniques to prospective brownfield site projects, including spatial demarcation and accounting in GIS databases and other parcel/property listings. This technological work subsidizes private industry's acquisition, remediation, and adaptive reuse of brownfield sites by optimizing data production for effective capital planning. Brownfield developers can also qualify for a range of subsidies, including tax increment financing (TIF), revolving funds (loans), trust funds (tax- or fee-based accounts), real estate trusts (private investments), tax credits and deferrals, or state grants. The 1997 Federal Taxpayer Relief Act enables developers to immediately reduce their taxable income by the cost of their eligible cleanup expenses. The law allows the costs of environmental cleanup to become fully deductible in the year they are incurred, thus help-

---

11. Dull and Wernstedt, "Land Recycling," 120.
12. Dull and Wernstedt, "Land Recycling," 119.

ing offset short-term cleanup costs.[13] To receive this incentive, the property earmarked for redevelopment must be located in a census tract area where more than 20 percent of the population resides below the mean poverty level and where 75 percent or more of the area's land is zoned for commercial or industrial use. Because these areas are often located within cities experiencing industrial manufacturing decline and devaluation, developers reap the benefits of reusing inexpensive, contaminated urban land to enjoy limited liability and high resale value.[14]

Such brownfield property redevelopment relies on assumptions about waste as a quantifiable and measurable object that can be separated and removed from land, or kept in place and contained to levels of risk deemed safe enough for a particular postcleanup end use. This way of thinking about waste maintains the illusion of a border between contamination and social life—a border on which capitalism's constant expansion and revival depends. Brownfield redevelopers strive to limit and contain their liability via property redevelopment schemes that rest on an underlying binary of waste/ society to establish the "conditions for a revival of profitability," predicated on a racialized logic of improvement.[15] Private developers are invited to invest in brownfields as an opportunity to turn a profit on converting economically unproductive land to public use. Brownfields deepen private sector engagement through amenities that boost private investment while immunizing investors from financial risk and biopolitical consequences. This process builds on long-standing practices that made—and maintained—environmentally degraded, economically divested, and racially marked lands.

13. Alan Berger, *Drosscape: Wasting Land in Urban America* (New York: Princeton Architectural Press, 2006), 70.

14. Berger, *Drosscape,* 74.

15. Jason W. Moore, "Ecology, Capital, and the Nature of Our Times: Accumulation and Crisis in the Capitalist World-Ecology," *Journal of World-Systems Research* 17, no. 1 (2011): 139.

Geographer Lindsey Dillon argues that the intimate proximity between environmental hazards and racialized bodies reveals that waste is one of the central modalities through which race has been lived in the twentieth century.[16] In turn, race has been and remains pivotal to signifying the "waste-ability of urban space."[17] As environmental justice activists and scholars across a range of fields attuned to critical studies of race have shown, race and waste have been articulated in specific geographical ways, leading to racialized health inequities and other disparities. Unequal social formations reproduce racial difference through spatial (de)valuation connected to the material presence of waste, as well as perceptions of "who" and "where" are unproductive and wastable. Property value is not the neutral measure of the worth of a particular piece of real estate but may be "better understood as the result of social and economic relations among places."[18] Jenna Loyd further explains that existing property systems, as well as the federal legislation, various authorities, and funding that support them, "build racial differentiation, class, and normative gender and sexual relations into the landscape."[19] Historically, for example, white single-family residential neighborhoods received low-interest loans for mortgages and high ratings in terms of their security value. Conversely, nonwhite land—often mixed use and adjacent to industry—was frequently redlined and considered an investment risk, subject to the racialized labels of "nuisance" and "blight." Couched in the supposedly impartial language of public health and planning, exclusionary zoning sequestered nonwhite people to contaminated,

16. Lindsey Dillon, "Race, Waste, and Space: Brownfield Redevelopment and Environmental Justice at the Hunters Point Shipyard," *Antipode* 46, no. 5 (2014): 1209.

17. Dillon, "Race, Waste, and Space," 1209.

18. Jenna Loyd, *Health Rights Are Civil Rights: Peace and Justice Activism in Los Angeles, 1963–1978* (Minneapolis: University of Minnesota Press, 2014), 28.

19. Loyd, *Health Rights,* 28.

vulnerable, and less desirable locations in an effort to protect white health and secure the value of whiteness as property.[20]

Brownfield redevelopments extend the legacy of property as an operation of racial capitalism and of pollution as colonialism.[21] Brownfield programs essentially maintain and expand practices that invested in public health for white communities and sanctioned contamination as part of historical racial segregation and disinvestment. They facilitate site conversions and cleanup remedies that minimize investor liability, thus often ensuring that contamination remains. Moreover, they facilitate land grabs and transfers through repossession, or "accumulation by degradation," where land is lost and gained because of its contamination.[22] Max Liboiron explains that "pollution is not only an exercise of colonial domination, it can also be part of its imperial expansion."[23] Scholars have warned that brownfield programs risk further entrenching "environmental apartheid" by implementing separate and unequal environmental standards across regions, particularly between inner cities and wealthier suburbs.[24] Grassroots activists and national environmental organizations have argued that "differential cleanup standards at brownfield sites could lead to a dangerous double standard and to a concentration of redeveloped sites in the inner cities where contamination has not been removed but rather contained on site"

20. Loyd, *Health Rights,* 28; David M. P. Freund, *Colored Property: State Policy and White Racial Politics in Suburban America* (Chicago: University of Chicago Press, 2007), 77–78, 118; Cheryl Harris, "Whiteness as Property," *Harvard Law Review* 106, no. 8 (1993): 1707–91.

21. Max Liboiron, *Pollution Is Colonialism* (Durham, N.C.: Duke University Press, 2021).

22. Leigh Johnson, "The Fearful Symmetry of Arctic Climate Change: Accumulation by Degradation," *Environment and Planning D: Society and Space* 28, no. 5 (2010): 828–47.

23. Max Liboiron, "Waste Colonialism," *Discard Studies,* November 1, 2018, https://discardstudies.com/2018/11/01/waste-colonialism/.

24. Georgette C. Poindexter, "Separate and Unequal: A Comment on the Urban Development Aspect of Brownfields Programs," *Fordham Urban Law Journal* 24, no. 1 (1996): 5.

to buffer life elsewhere.[25] Furthermore, brownfields can serve as a technocratic instrument to determine whose bodies and communities can be wasted. Brownfields facilitate contingent determinations of value about whose lives and whose health matter and whose racially marked bodies and futures do not.

Brownfield programs pose significant problems for public participation, intensifying the ongoing racial ordering of land and territorial control as well as further curtailing minority participation in governance. Heightened reliance on private investments and private property controls to address residual site hazards results in decisions about future land use that increasingly depend on proprietary information that is unavailable to the public. Private investors who encourage brownfield redevelopments may seek to curtail or eliminate public input in order to limit liability and facilitate faster turnover of the site, even as citizen groups demand a say in the recycling of land. Deed restrictions enshrine private ownership of property, leaving the public at risk, all while brownfield projects avow goals of improving environmental health. The economic calculus of brownfield redevelopment restricts, even obstructs, a knowing and involved public. Brownfield developers receive state-certified liability releases for cleanups in the form of covenants not to sue after cleanup, no-further-action agreements, gag order clauses in property sales documents, and so forth. In addition to freeing developers from any further responsibility for adverse environmental and biopolitical effects, the state agrees that it will not require or impose additional cleanup requirements at a later date if acceptable cleanup standards are implemented.

Such standards are tied to a risk-based understanding of anticipated land use that extends waste colonialism. Because different end uses of the site require distinct tiers of remediation standards, land recycling efforts enlist remediation options that range from minor remediation needed for limited human contact, such as fu-

25. Wernstedt and Hersh, "Through a Lens Darkly," 160.

ture use as a parking lot, to widespread waste removal from the site or on-site underground waste containment. Developers typically remove the upper level of soil and replace it with clean soil placed atop an impervious cap meant to prevent exposure to arsenic, lead, chromium, or any other remaining contamination capable of reaching the surface. In some cases, engineered systems may be constructed to pump out contaminated groundwater or to capture noxious odors. Governance of the remaining on-site contamination hinges on what are considered safe levels of risk according to the type of land reuse and ongoing hazards. The process essentially locks communities into a future of permissible contamination tied to a specific site use with little to no public discussion. Moreover, local governments often have little incentive to restrict land use and impose controls, few resources, and limited financial capacity to monitor or enforce controls; in many cases, they face strong political pressure for unrestricted use of a site.[26] The overall managerial ontology at work fosters some futures and eclipses others by assimilating what la paperson characterizes as "the life worlds of land, air, water, plants and animals, and Indigenous peoples [that] are reconfigured into natural resources, chattel, and waste: statuses whose capitalist 'value' does not depend on whether they are living or dead but only on their fungibility and disposability."[27]

Brownfield programs wed environmental risk reduction to economic development as part of the broader integration of economic priorities in federal hazardous waste policy and the cycle of land dispossession/repossession that characterizes racial capitalism and ongoing U.S. settler-colonial property governance. This raises equity issues. Many brownfield sites lie in minority communities, where lower-income people have been relocated to devalued land or left underserved for decades. Yet studies have found "negative

26. Wernstedt and Hersh, "Through a Lens Darkly," 172.
27. La paperson, *A Third University Is Possible* (Minneapolis: University of Minnesota Press, 2017), 14–15; Liboiron, *Pollution Is Colonialism,* 65.

correlations between the proportions of local populations that are nonwhite or low-income and the likelihood of receiving an award" for brownfield redevelopment.[28] Contrary to the EPA's explicit commitments to equity with respect to land revitalization, applicants from localities with higher concentrations of poverty and higher numbers of self-identified nonwhites have been historically less likely to receive an EPA brownfields award.[29] The brownfield framework assembles a property frontier that aggregates and homogenizes a diverse array of land types labeled "underutilized potential"—a category akin to the settler-colonial ideology of *terra nullius* (empty land).[30] This process renders such lands commensurable, marking them as available for redevelopment projects with the potential to generate a high return thanks to financial subsidies and liability caps. To revive conditions of profitability, each brownfield site is treated as discrete territory, regardless of regional patterns of disinvestment and environmental decline.[31] For cities or regions under conditions of austerity, brownfields become part of the austerity policy arsenal directed at distressed areas for environmental violations that are the result of larger-scale processes of wasting and devaluing. The spatial fetishism of the brownfield enables city officials and developers to target and intervene in delineated properties, and in doing so, they negate current site uses and even blame existing communities for having underutilized or environmentally degraded the land.

Brownfield programs support the racialized operations of the private property system by justifying land dispossession of areas of actual or perceived contamination and uncertain environmental hazards in terms of risks to health. The symptoms of a neighborhood's systemic neglect, including degraded infrastructure, environmental hazards, and racialized health inequities, can serve as

28. Dull and Wernstedt, "Land Recycling," 119.
29. Dull and Wernstedt, "Land Recycling," 134.
30. Nunn, "Toxic Encounters," 1337.
31. Loyd, *Health Rights,* 30.

justification for exercising eminent domain based on the argument that it is a public necessity. Under the proviso of public improvement, cities and their favored developers can point to the legacies of structural-institutional-environmental racism and any number of conditions resulting from the nexus of race, waste, and space—from sewer floodplain hazards and high quantities of lead in water systems to asthma rates linked to industrial pollution—as a rationale for the removal of low-income residents and communities of color from land, homes, and the ability to secure safe, stable living.

The brownfield framework draws on the long-standing policy discourse of "blight" as racially marked land that legitimates eminent domain and seizure in the name of public use. Definitions of what constitutes public use have typically been left to each state, and the U.S. Supreme Court has made increasingly broader determinations over the years.[32] In 2005, the Supreme Court ruled that cities may legally seize private property for "economic development" even if that property is not blighted, essentially sanctioning any city seizure of private land that could receive higher property tax revenues with a new or different public use. The ruling supports urban renewal practices that have, over decades, tied the laudable objective of creating healthy cities and affordable housing to the amorphous discourse of blight and its racialized stigma. For example, the Housing Act of 1949 provided the legislative basis for the American urban renewal program that was tasked with supplying an adequate living environment for every American family. Instead, it became tethered to the objective of removing urban blight. Urban renewal advocates enlisted metaphors of plant pathology and medical disease to provide a scientific basis for blight. By elevating blight into a destructive and contagious urban disease, renewal advocates stretched the application of public use as a requirement of eminent

32. Colin M. McNiece, "A Public Use for the Dirty Side of Economic Development: Finding Common Ground between Kelo and Hathcock for Collateral Takings in Brownfield Redevelopment," *Roger Williams University Law Review* 12, no. 1 (2006): 230–36.

domain, with property rights reconceptualized so that so-called blighted properties "were considered less worthy of the full bundle of rights recognized by American law."[33] Blight served as a useful rhetorical device to reorganize property ownership according to productive and unproductive land uses. Although it was purportedly a neutral, scientific understanding of urban decline, it was used to warrant the removal of Black and other minority residents from parts of the city.[34] Determinations of blight sanctioned massive land clearance and removal of BIPOC populations from land deemed to be deteriorated, dysfunctional, poor, and unproductive. Federal resources underwrote the redevelopment costs. In Rachel Weber's depiction, "like teams of surgeons, city government removed the concentrations of blight while the federal government assumed the role of the insurance company, absorbing the costs of demolition and land preparation."[35]

Brownfields extend this genealogy of subsidized land appropriation and redevelopment. Local and state governments use the power to take private property based on blight—amplified by the ambiguous, elastic definitions of public use found in brownfield programs—to accelerate the gentrification and displacement already affecting low-income BIPOC communities. Cities are designating property as blighted not necessarily because it exhibits conditions of toxicity but rather because the city views the property as unproductive from a tax revenue perspective.[36] The preemptive exercise of eminent domain to reorganize urban land—whether to eliminate potential pollution or to support public use in cases where environmental health is not even a primary concern—takes on the logic of providing a public benefit for the "good of the city."[37] This

33. Pritchett, "Public Menace," 4.

34. Pritchett, "Public Menace," 6, 18.

35. Rachel Weber, "Extracting Value from the City: Neoliberalism and Urban Redevelopment," *Antipode* 34, no. 3 (2002): 527.

36. Berger, *Drosscape*, 75.

37. Pritchett, "Public Menace," 26.

expansion of eminent domain legalizes the condemnation of property and its transfer to private parties under the public use clause, where assessments of the state of urban infrastructure determine that "this land is too good for these people" and could be put to a better use.[38] Municipalities and local governments can opportunistically define blight according to their own city or regional planning interests, especially to generate fast revenue through commercial and retail projects.[39]

Scenarios wherein an urban renewal authority or city agency attempts to declare eminent domain on a property in order to attract big box stores have grown rapidly in areas that are experiencing economic decline. The home improvement chain Home Depot actively seeks to develop store locations on urban brownfield sites, receiving tax breaks and remediating contaminated sites to lay vast parking lots in cities as disparate as Honolulu and Pittsburgh. Walmart similarly pursues brownfield redevelopment: the Denver Urban Renewal Authority targeted the largest pan-Asian grocery store in the city, along with a strip mall of popular Asian restaurants, to grant Walmart $10 million in tax subsidies to redevelop the site.[40] The city's eviction and redevelopment plan was only thwarted after a lengthy community petition process. In the case of Emeryville, California, the city took control of a hallowed shell mound of the Ohlone people through eminent domain proceedings that considered the site merely as postindustrial urban wasteland and taxable city property.[41] Emeryville, dubbed a poster child for brownfield redevelopment, conducted urban renewal of this sacred ground by digging into the massive human-made mound of shells, tools,

38. Pritchett, "Public Menace," 21, quoting sociologist Scott Greer's 1965 assessment of the urban renewal program.

39. McNiece, "Public Use," 230–36.

40. Berger, *Drosscape,* 75.

41. Rick DelVecchio, "Urban Renewal Atop Sacred Past/Ohlone Protest Emeryville Project," *SFGate,* November 20, 2002, https://www.sfgate.com/bayarea/article/Urban-renewal-atop-sacred-past-Ohlone-protest-2752176.php.

bowls, animal bones, and human burials created over the course of 2,500 years to construct the Bay Street retail and entertainment complex. The shell mound, which once stood more than thirty feet high and three hundred feet long, had been desecrated by earlier land conversions, including the occupation of the site by an amusement park and dance hall, followed by heavy industry in the 1920s that left vats of toxic chemicals and polluted soils from a defunct pigment plant.[42] Emeryville's redevelopment agency subsequently stripped the ground of toxic dirt and hired a developer to create the Main Street commercial village that is now hailed nationally as a model of urban land reclamation. On Black Fridays, Ohlone activists and protestors converge near the intersection of Shellmound Street and Ohlone Way to honor the site's significance, demand land rematriation, and remind shoppers that they are standing on a living cemetery—a cemetery where reportedly one hundred human burials were taken from the metered parking lot behind Victoria's Secret, and several other hundred were reburied on site in an unmarked grave anchoring the mixed-use development.[43]

While the EPA now acknowledges that brownfields may be Tribal lands, it remains unclear whether brownfield programs will conduct land reparations for Native communities and descendants. The

---

42. Rob Arias, "2005 'Shellmound' Documentary Exposes the Truth Behind, and Under, Bay Street Development," *E'ville Eye*, January 15, 2014, https://evilleeye.com/history/2005-shellmound-documentary-exposes-the-truth-behind-and-under-bay-street-developement/.

43. Seven hundred bodies were previously taken from the site to the University of California, Berkeley. Allison Griner, "'On My Ancestors' Remains': The Fight for Sacred Lands," *Aljazeera,* December 16, 2019, https://www.aljazeera.com/features/2019/12/16/on-my-ancestors-remains-the-fight-for-sacred-lands; Sara Zaske, "Emeryville Officials Will Honor Ohlone Site before Destroying It," *East Bay Express,* May 18, 2001, https://www.eastbayexpress.com/oakland/emeryville-officials-will-honor-ohlone-site-before-destroying-it/Content?oid=1065448. Urban Indigenous women–led Sogorea Te' Land Trust (https://sogoreate-landtrust.org/) reclaims the shell mounds and unceded Lisjan territory of Huchiun (known as Oakland, Berkeley, Alameda, Piedmont, Emeryville, and Albany, California).

productivity imperative of the property system—and the broader functioning of property law as a U.S. settler-colonial technology, with all of the knowledge and financial institutions that support it[44]—actively organizes and maintains the *social death of land* to the extent that in Emeryville, a strip mall now contains ancestral burials and toxic waste in a still-active cycle of repudiation and erasure.[45] Essentially, brownfield policy and financial instruments create an ad hoc property frontier of "wastelands." As a result of the uncertain presence of waste, contaminated land is always potential in terms of economic viability; it provides an opportunity for future surplus value production.[46] Brownfields promise higher returns thanks to their higher stakes—as long as measures and rewards are in place to mitigate investor risk related to the unknown extent of contamination.

This utility for economic productivity is a colonial way of understanding contaminated land as a wasteland with potential. It works within the structural context of U.S. settler colonialism and racial capitalism—namely "the systematic extraction of value organized through racial hierarchy" and its accompanying racialization of space.[47] Physical contamination of land articulates

44. Paperson, *Third University*, 4.

45. I use Orlando Patterson's framework of social death to emphasize land seizures that underpin property in the United States and the colonial fantasy of land as unmarked rather than a politicized/violent set of relations between property owners and others. Orlando Patterson, *Slavery and Social Death: A Comparative Study* (Cambridge, Mass.: Harvard University Press, 1982).

46. Max Liboiron, Manuel Tironi, and Nerea Calvillo, "Toxic Politics: Acting in a Permanently Polluted World," *Social Studies of Science* 48, no. 3 (2018): 331–49.

47. Danielle M. Purifoy and Louise Seamster, "Creative Extraction: Black Towns in White Space," *Environment and Planning D: Society and Space* 39, no. 1 (2020): 51; Cedric J. Robinson, *Black Marxism: The Making of the Black Radical Tradition* (Chapel Hill, NC: University of North Carolina Press, 1983). Here I use "colonial" and not "settler-colonial" to refer to the property enclosure process pertaining to multiple forms of colonialism, not only the specific settler-colonial project that is the United States.

with colonial notions of improvement and productivity to delineate the brownfield as a new enclosure: postindustrial land with (real or perceived) contamination available for development projects and property renewal.[48] Historically, land uses that procured maximum economic value were considered proper to civilization; conversely, land or wilderness that had not yet been drawn into colonial or national development capitalist relations were perceived as wasteful or as waste.[49] Settler-colonial enclosure sought to reframe land as a resource by enacting a way of seeing the world based on a logic of expropriation and the economic right "to realize the maximum productive potential of all things, at all times, and in all ways."[50] Extending this morality of economic use and its opposite as waste, brownfields policy converts pollution's stubborn presence/excess into mere financial, legal, and technical matters that support the settler-colonial logic of "public reuse" of land and facilitate the racialized targeting of BIPOC spaces through an ongoing cycle of toxicity.

Brownfield conversions often orchestrate a violent feedback loop of land repossession as dispossession that reenacts frontier logics— or, as Sharon Stein explains, "The U.S. state's genocidal efforts to conquer the literal frontier helped to solidify a colonial template of state-facilitated capital accumulation that is premised on the conquest of a perpetual frontier."[51] Waste frontier offers blank space to facilitate land grabs and extraction. It might be a state's takeover of land as new territory, or it might be using land as a containment

48. Brenna Bhandar, *Colonial Lives of Property: Law, Land, and Racial Regimes of Ownership* (Durham, N.C.: Duke University Press, 2018).

49. Liboiron, "Waste Colonialism," discussing Jessie Goldstein, "*Terra Economica:* Waste and the Production of Enclosed Nature," *Antipode* 45, no. 2 (2013): 357–75.

50. Goldstein, "*Terra Economica,*" 371, 368.

51. Sharon Stein, "A Colonial History of the Higher Education Present: Rethinking Land-grant Institutions Through Processes of Accumulation and Relations of Conquest," *Critical Studies in Education* 61, no. 2 (2020): 213.

space "to externalize the toxic burdens."[52] Spatial demarcation and GIS-based accounting of land supports private redevelopment within the property market by producing surfaces of transfer, seizure, and exchange that allow for the burial, monitoring, and forgetting of waste. Such an approach makes ambiguous the technical inventorying of land with predatory targeting of marginalized communities; such an approach also facilitates the ongoing denial of the environmental harms perpetrated by settler-colonial, racialized land practices and occupation of space. By affixing contamination on site and treating space as unrelational and accounted for in database entries and GIS-layered renderings, brownfield programs disembed the land market from material conditions of waste and its racialized geographies. Because brownfield programs make contamination legible as a frontier for high returns with limited liability for uncertain toxicity, there is no incentive to inventory the history of site hazards and waste as a ruin of racist disinvestment and uneven geographies of wealth and poverty. Instead, brownfields maintain internal colonization territorially and fiscally through conquest of devalued landscapes seen to have potential—a determination that enables settlers to know city space as theirs, with them as the managers and rightful inhabitants of public or civilized space.[53] With the entire property system built on stolen Native land, this brownfield frontier supports renewed rounds of forced removal, occupation, and erasure of BIPOC inhabitants in the name of redevelopment, thereby amplifying the need to address brownfields as a deeply historical, spatial, and cross-generational racial justice issue.

While brownfield policy remains invested in the property system, the redevelopment methodology is not wholly determined by such frontier logics. Indeed, it has been instrumentalized to

52. Purifoy and Seamster, "Creative Extraction," 56, 52.

53. Karina Czyzewski, "Colonialism as a Broader Social Determinant of Health," *International Indigenous Policy Journal* 2, no. 1 (2011): 2, drawing on Sherene Razack, "Violence against First Nations: On Ongoing Colonialism," paper presented at University of British Columbia, Okanagan, October 22, 2008.

foster more community sovereignty and land reciprocity in response to pollution, devaluation, and other social determinants of health that become the pretext for displacement. Brownfield projects that reframe land revitalization in terms of health equity and environmental stewardship, for example, represent the potential to advance goals of enhancing care for BIPOC communities and rearranging historical geographies of segregation and disinvestment.[54] Both the EPA and the Agency for Toxic Substances and Disease Registry recognize an important aspect of land reuse for public health improvement beyond economic development.[55] A form of brownfield project called healthfields holds the promise of reframing land revitalization as an ongoing public health effort involving community stewardship of bodies of land and human health. This U.S. land reuse policy also seeks to ameliorate medical scarcity in underserved BIPOC communities and to work across the U.S. biomedical divide that separates bodily health and clinic-based acute care from environmental conditions.

Healthfields are brownfields ostensibly used for health purposes, such as health care centers, grocery stores, farmers markets, green spaces, and in some cases affordable housing. The "EPA Brownfields to Healthfields" website defines healthfields as an "economic development strategy that has served lower income families living in environmentally overburdened neighborhoods."[56] An EPA story map detailing healthfields through visual media and textual narrative shows that healthfields increase local access to health care and community clinics, parks and open space, food access, and housing—

54. Land reciprocity and reparations, however, remain essential to decolonizing brownfields and settler environmentalism.

55. U.S. EPA, "Incorporating Health Monitoring Activities into an EPA Brownfields Grant," EPA 560-F-18-187 (2018), https://www.epa.gov/sites/production/files/2015-09/documents/finalphandbffact.pdf.

56. U.S. EPA, "Brownfields to Healthfields," accessed November 7, 2022, http://www.arcgis.com/apps/MapSeries/index.html?appid=76cd82c-0c167480799ab9e6f6f144e36.

all through cleanup and reuse of former brownfield sites.[57] The term "healthfield" first cropped up around the year 2014 in Florida, and it has since been popularized by Miles Ballogg, the director for brownfields and economic development for Cardno TBE, an engineering consulting firm self-described as a professional infrastructure and environmental services company. Ballogg and Cardno have been leaders of healthfield projects and advocacy in Florida, but there are also prominent examples in places like McComb, Mississippi, and Los Angeles, California.[58] The EPA report "Improving Public Health in Brownfields Communities" details the benefits of healthfield redevelopment: "In addition to the restoration of blighted, idle land and the removal of contamination, residents now have improved access to health care, new jobs, and local economic engines that leverage additional improvements and enhance quality of life."[59] The literature on healthfields emphasizes that brownfield law provides local governments and brownfield communities with the opportunity to link land revitalization with public health through provisions that allow local governments to spend up to 10 percent of their grants to conduct health monitoring of populations in sites where people may be exposed to hazardous substances and what is termed "legacy contamination." Frequently cited healthfield projects range from asthma surveillance mapping of children linked to school-based health programs to the conversion of defunct gas stations into parks, farmers markets, and health services centers.

The healthfield program debuted with the Willa Carson Health and Wellness Center in Clearwater, Florida. This case was driven by

57. U.S. EPA, "From Brownfields to Healthfields," 2019, https://epa.maps.arcgis.com/apps/Cascade/index.html?appid=fa7b68b3075a-4340970b1e5c00c76cf4.

58. Ronda Kaysen, "Health Centers Find Opportunity in Brownfields," *New York Times,* December 11, 2012, http://www.nytimes.com/2012/12/12/realestate/commercial/health-centers-find-opportunity-in-brownfields.html?_r=1&.

59. U.S. EPA, "Improving Public Health in Brownfields Communities," EPA-560-F-07-253, January 2008, https://archive.epa.gov/socal/web/pdf/public_health08.pdf.

Willa Carson herself, who had already been operating a community health care center and wanted to raise enough money to open a more permanent facility for a free clinic to service residents of the city's North Greenwood community. A derelict gas station was deemed an ideal place for the health center thanks to its central community location. Using EPA and state brownfield program funds, four underground storage tanks and 450 tons of contaminated soil were removed from the property. The city then leased the property to the nonprofit clinic—which Carson had previously operated out of two refurbished apartments—for thirty years at the rate of $1 per year.[60] Opening in 2001, the Willa Carson Health Resource Center provides free health care predominantly to the surrounding African American community and is operated on donations and grants with the help of a volunteer workforce.[61]

Another brownfield conversion that fulfills critical needs and greatly improved medical access for local residents is the Johnnie Ruth Clarke Health Center at the historic Mercy Hospital in St. Petersburg, Florida. Beset with petroleum contamination from a former cab company as well as hazardous waste from the African American hospital that operated on the grounds for over forty years, this healthfield project sought to install a new community-run health services center in the tradition of Jim Crow–era African American medical activism, providing residents with immediate access to health care and an economic anchor for further neighborhood redevelopment. Funded with a $3.75 million U.S. Department of Health and Human Services grant and $463,000 U.S. Housing and Urban Development Community Development Block Grant funds, the center's construction began in 2003 and included the preser-

60. U.S. EPA, "Improving Public Health."
61. Miles Ballogg in partnership with U.S. EPA and the City of Tampa, Florida, "'Healthfields': Improving Access to Healthcare through Brownfields Redevelopment," paper presented at EPA Brownfields 2013 conference, May 16, 2013, http://www.georgiaenet.com/wp-content/uploads/2015/01/23MilesBallogg.pdf (access via the 2013 Georgia Environmental Conference).

vation of the 1923 historic hospital building and a new museum dedicated to the history of African American medicine in Pinellas County.[62] The Johnnie Ruth Clarke Health Center foregrounds the potential of healthfields to convert legacies of health disparities tied to racial segregation into geographies of justice based on community-driven health services and land revitalization. The site is a brownfield partly because of the past lack of infrastructure for medical waste removal—what an EPA Brownfields conference presentation described as "abandoned historic African American Hospital environmental issues."[63]

The development of the health center at this Jim Crow–era hospital brings more community health services to an underserved area, but it does not significantly alter the spatialization of waste and racial inequity. The emphasis of brownfield programs, and by extension healthfields, on environmental cleanup standards and land futures allied to property productivity potentially means that significant but uncertain contamination remains. In this sense, healthfields represent a contradiction: such programs may offer badly needed health services, but they risk reentrenching health disparities stemming from historic segregation, environmental racism, and waste colonialism. Healthfields may only superficially address the land's hazards, thus ensuring exposure to contamination continues. This negative outcome of healthfields may be further intensified by the type of healthfield developed: the broad definition includes corporate packaged-food box stores, for-profit health service chains (often referred to as Medicaid mills), or pharmaceutical manufacturing, the latter being an especially well-known polluting industry. Healthfields may also support the growth of nonprofit philanthrocapitalist medical surveillance, as well as the installation of high-end hospital zones that exploit devalued land and the poor communities that live there while receiving tax breaks for their

62. U.S. EPA, "Improving Public Health." In 2019, the nonprofit occupant community health centers of Pinellas spent $3.95 million to move to a new headquarters and renovate Johnnie Ruth Clarke.
63. Ballogg, "Healthfields."

provision of humanitarian services. Even as healthfields create an opportunity to bring health care to underserved areas and rearrange historical geographies of hospital locations that arose along lines of segregation rather than epidemiological need, they also potentially serve as "Jim Crow tax shelters" that thrive on blight renewal—what la paperson refers to as the "ghetto land pedagogy" of settler colonialism.[64]

Thus, while healthfields to some degree show that "land can be polluted and still foster good land relations,"[65] the continued prioritizing of property values and an environmentally inequitable and extractive logic incentivizes development projects that target vulnerable populations; it justifies ongoing land grabs under the banner of environmental health. Planting parks, farmers markets, or other environmental amenities as trickle-down benefits to local health-stricken communities can intensify gentrification and entrench geographies of waste and race by "greenwashing" displacement. Healthfield projects tether the reuse of brownfield sites to health purposes—namely local access to health care clinics—yet can function to greenwash austerity, poverty, and contamination. In so doing, healthfields can perpetuate ill health. The initiative offers tax breaks and lowers cleanup standards and liability to health projects that remedy toxic blight: even as healthfield programs create an opportunity for community-oriented land remedies, they also spur the growth of extractive development projects that exploit devalued land and do not necessarily give local communities a seat at the table of economic planning and governance.

This critical speculation on healthfields underscores how brownfield policy organizes a new waste frontier that expands the ra-

64. Paperson argues that "the ghetto serves as an interior frontier to be laid waste in order to renew." La paperson, "A Ghetto Land Pedagogy: An Antidote for Settler Environmentalism," *Environmental Education Research* 20, no. 1 (2014): 116. My term "Jim Crow tax shelters" refers to the tax-exempt, nonprofit shadow of the state—humanitarian philanthrocapitalist organizations and services—that maintain a financial color line.

65. Liboiron, *Pollution Is Colonialism*, 22.

tionale for and application of eminent domain to the racialized logics of blight. Brownfield site conversions generate value through contingent determinations of productivity and public use; they implement waste remediation and land renewal in ways that intensify the everyday environmental degradation, disinvestment, displacement, and poverty experienced by BIPOC communities. The example of healthfields raises further questions about the targeting of contaminated land located in BIPOC communities who suffer from the presence of waste and who are underserved by health care providers. The healthfields initiative aims to convert targeted areas into hospitals, wellness centers, and grocery stores, offering tax breaks that invite "green health" projects. Brownfields/ healthfields promise an ad hoc postindustrial frontier that makes contaminated land available for cleanup and revitalization, and that can serve as an important means for generating liquidity in cash-strapped urban areas with small tax bases.[66] The attendant discourse of blight claims that brownfield redevelopment enhances public health; in practice, however, such redevelopment is structured to lower cleanup standards and reduce liability. The two cases of brownfield and healthfield—and their respective goals of boosting the economy and improving public health—show how blight designation can be used to gentrify inner-city areas or arbitrarily secure more profitable site usage, and how health service installations may paradoxically entrench health inequities, economic injustices, and environmental hazards stemming from segregation and previous rounds of land seizure.

Examining this policy environment and set of practices provides important context for the health sector's formal role in land valuation and perpetuating racial inequities in health. Brownfields provide insights on the U.S. property frontier—its articulations of waste and race tied to determinations of productive versus unproductive

66. Richard Briffault, "The Most Popular Tool: Tax Increment Financing and the Political Economy of Local Government," *University of Chicago Law Review* 77, no. 1 (2010): 72.

land use—and liberal regimes of value, such as the moralistic discourse of blight, that justify land grabs and displacement as environmental improvement and public health benefit. In the next chapter, I utilize this framework to critically review the land development policies and practices of large nonprofit hospitals, excavating the policy terrain known as Eds and Meds. The discussion considers how these nonprofit institutions actively foster medical brownfields: they maintain the toxic open door of the property system and racially uneven urban regional health care; facilitate eminent domain in territorial and fiscal ways while declaring community benefits, local development, sustainability, and even racial justice; and build urban biomedical complexes by extracting from the environmental and economic livelihoods of BIPOC communities.

2. Hospital Growth Machines and Colonizing Brownfields

BIOMEDICAL INSTITUTIONS operate on land and engage in territorial strategies, such as property acquisitions. Hospitals in particular pursue development goals that actively shape space, including both local place-based investments and transnational infrastructure. The health sector interfaces with and facilitates the racially inequitable property system. Biomedical institutions inevitably participate in legacies of segregation and oppression that are spatially manifested in urban regional economies—in the arrangement of residences, work life, infrastructures, public services, and financial priorities. Redlining, to return to that example, secured spaces for white investment and subsidized white life through the exclusive location of and restricted access to safe environments and health services, such as hospitals. Conversely, this urban land management practice limited nonwhite and poor people's ability to secure financial resources necessary for building wealth; it also contained them in undesirable areas of the inner-city or industrial periphery. U.S. land policies have denied economic and health resources to a significant portion of the population even as, contradictorily, public health and civic-oriented ideals, from sanitation to land revitalization, have been used to frame and maintain the racialized property system.

U.S. urban policies have historically driven health policy toward property-oriented growth with racially oppressive effects.

Examples include the institutionalized segregation of hospitals in terms of location and access at the regional and citywide level; and the highly localized experiences of medical and food scarcity, insurance discrimination, and other pervasive forms of medical redlining.[1] Hospitals contribute to this complex geography of health and racial disparity in many ways, including their role as historic land-grab institutions and land developers, propelled by urban policies that funnel capital into real estate. Hospitals and public health have featured prominently in efforts to target land for redevelopment, exacerbating segregation and displacing residents of minority neighborhoods to facilitate the expansion of high-end service industries in urban cores where manufacturing has declined. As I explained in chapter 1, land has consistently been made available for redevelopment through colonizing discourses of blight, public improvement, and health tied to economic productivity, which erase or denigrate nonwhite spaces and communities to prime land for seizure. Biomedical institutions participate actively in the racializing and fiscalizing of land, a process that creates a medical brownfield frontier for urban redevelopment projects with privatizing and profit-making aims often couched in civic ideals. The land-grant legacy of stolen Native land to support agriculture and rural area development became a dominant paradigm for urban land-grant universities and urban development partnerships involving hospitals, thereby highlighting land dispossession as the base of the U.S. property system's financial mechanisms and civic notions of public goods or benefits.[2]

1. Vernellia Randall, "Institutional Racism in U.S. Health Care," Institute on Race, Health Care and the Law, University of Dayton School of Law, 1993, 2008, https://academic.udayton.edu/health/07humanrights/racial01c.htm.

2. Steven J. Diner, "The Land-Grant Analogy and the American Urban University: An Historical Analysis," *Metropolitan Universities* 23, no. 3 (2012): 61–77; Robert Lee and Tristan Ahtone, "Land-Grab Universities," *High Country News,* March 30, 2020, https://www.hcn.org/issues/52.4/indigenous-affairs-education-land-grab-universities; Sharon Stein,

Hospitals have long served as instruments of urban renewal and economic growth; they enhance property values and raise revenues. According to urban health historian Guian A. McKee, federal programs motivated the expansion and modernization of urban hospitals during the post–World War II period both directly, through subsidies, and indirectly, through tax expenditures.[3] These public policies supported the physical growth of urban health care institutions and their research activities, with hospitals increasingly replacing factories as the urban economic core.[4] Hospitals not only provided medical care but also took on the increasingly important role of anchoring postindustrial cities.[5] The Hill-Burton loan and grant program, passed in 1946 as the Hospital Survey and Construction Act, offered federal matching grants for the construction of new hospitals and nursing homes, essentially covering 10 percent of the construction costs.[6] Initially slated for rural areas, a 1964 amendment permitted the program to issue grants to modernize existing hospitals regardless of previous per capita bed limitations. The Housing Act of 1949 offered local governments a "write-down" subsidy that covered two-thirds of the cost of assembling and clearing blighted land for "predominantly residential" redevelopment.[7] Section 112 of the 1959 amendments gave hospitals the opportunity to take advantage of the federal

---

"Confronting the Racial-Colonial Foundations of U.S. Higher Education," *Journal for the Study of Postsecondary and Tertiary Education* 3 (2018): 77–98.

3. Guian A. McKee, "Health-Care Policy as Urban Policy: Hospitals and Community Development in the Postindustrial City," Working Paper 2010-10, Center for Community Development Investments, December 2010, https://www.frbsf.org/community-development/publications/working-papers/2010/december/health-care-policy-urban/, 5.

4. Guian A. McKee, "The Hospital City in an Ethnic Enclave: Tufts–New England Medical Center, Boston's Chinatown, and the Urban Political Economy of Health Care," *Journal of Urban History* 42, no. 2 (2016): 260.

5. Davarian L. Baldwin, *In the Shadow of the Ivory Tower: How Universities Are Plundering Our Cities* (New York: Bold Type, 2021), 7–12.

6. McKee, "Health-Care Policy," 5.

7. This act is popularly known as the U.S. urban renewal program.

subsidy; it presumed that urban renewal conducted by and for private institutional purposes aided the public good.[8] Once legislation opened the door for urban renewal funding with no requirement for housing, medical facilities launched expansion projects and actively participated in what Malini Ranganathan frames as the "conjoined processes of racialized property making and property taking," linking medical planning offices to citywide renewal processes.[9] By 1964, U.S. urban renewal projects involved seventy-five hospitals, including major urban medical centers such as Johns Hopkins University Hospital in Baltimore and the Detroit Medical Center.[10] The University of Alabama displaced over 10,000 Black residents of Birmingham to raise its now highly acclaimed medical research campus during this period.[11] The paradigm of land-grant institutions evolved into a moral geography of civic duty to appropriate land to "solve" city problems.

Cities welcomed real estate projects in the health sector because they could claim these expenditures as local grants-in-aid matched by federal support at a 2:1 ratio, beyond which local funds could be banked as credits for future urban renewal projects.[12] Aided by the moralizing discourse of blight that confounded public and private responsibility, select well-established urban hospitals benefited from funds to renovate buildings and inaugurate new centers within a health care system that remained largely exclusionary. Cities could apply banked hospital expansion credits toward expensive downtown redevelopment plans. Hospitals, nursing homes, and other medical clinics would also enter into real estate ventures in the expanding white suburbs, with subsidized new facilities that

8. McKee, "Hospital City," 262.

9. Malini Ranganathan, "Thinking with Flint: Racial Liberalism and the Roots of an American Water Tragedy," *Capitalism Nature Socialism* 27 (2016), https://doi.org/10.1080/10455752.2016.1206583, 6.

10. McKee, "Health-Care Policy," 7.

11. Bobby M. Wilson, "Racial Segregation Trends in Birmingham, Alabama," *Southeastern Geographer* 25, no. 1 (1985): 32–33.

12. McKee, "Health-Care Policy," 5–6.

contributed to the racialized arrangement of urban regions. Even after federal support shifted from direct spending to loans, with hospitals financing a greater percentage of construction through debt financing as opposed to raising capital, the government continued its subsidies by guaranteeing hospital mortgages.[13] The Federal Housing Administration, well known for its role in promoting suburbanization and subsidized white flight, buffered massive hospital expansions and growth through a mortgage insurance program by which hospitals saved millions in debt service because of reduced interest rates.

This brief gloss of an earlier period of urban renewal affecting U.S. cities underscores how cities channel capital into local real estate assets through health care institutions. More broadly, it indicates the fiscalization of municipal land use decisions, which, for local governments, increases the value of taxable resources in order to raise revenues without rate hikes.[14] Faced with the political imperative to build and the capitalist demand for liquidity, local states have developed mechanisms that discursively code and order the meaning of place to make the built environment more responsive to the investment criteria of real estate capital.[15] Tax increment financing emerged as one such strategy. Cities historically used TIF to raise local contributions, which were required by the urban renewal program to obtain federal matching funds for redevelopment projects. TIF entailed designating a quasi-public development authority and territorially defining a submunicipal area, thus delineating blighted properties as special tax increment districts where municipalities would fund projects up front by pledging future property tax revenues as security for current borrowing.[16] The portion (increment) of taxes generated as a result of the rede-

13. McKee, "Hospital City," 263.

14. Briffault, "Most Popular Tool," 86.

15. Weber, "Extracting Value," 520, 524.

16. Rachel Weber, "Selling City Futures: The Financialization of Urban Redevelopment Policy," *Economic Geography* 86, no. 3 (2010): 258.

velopment would, in theory, finance the improvements. In this way, cities obtained capital by turning rights to their own heterogeneous property tax base into standardized tradeable assets.[17] TIFs fortified physical infrastructure, land acquisition, site clearance, and other programs that reduce a developer's capital costs, as cities gambled on future appreciation in the value of land and buildings within the demarcated geographic area. By codifying select areas as blighted as a precondition for investment, TIFs justified land grabs under the proviso of future returns and economic benefits. This fiscal-territorial strategy of development is now widely used by local governments as an all-purpose tool for financing public investment. TIF-backed projects can be found in suburbs and edge-city interchanges in addition to the inner city.[18]

Recent decades of urban redevelopment projects have implemented TIFs to revitalize downtowns within the former industrial core of cities. Between 1992 and 2007, the U.S. Department of Housing and Urban Development made nearly $80 billion available for inner-city redevelopment of underutilized public housing and postindustrial blight.[19] When property values decline because of environmental contamination, cities may freeze the value at the reduced level and consider any restored property value as the increment on which to finance the cleanup. As previously discussed, brownfield policies routinely involve TIFs, tax breaks, and other incentives to redevelop contaminated land. Brownfields codify a postindustrial frontier of available contaminated land. The remediation of this frontier provides the material basis for entrepreneurial forms of property redevelopment and waste management. The discourse of blight allows brownfield policy and practice to claim public health benefits, all while restricting liability and lowering cleanup standards tied to "productive" future land uses.

17. Weber, "Selling City Futures," 258.
18. Briffault, "Most Popular Tool," 71–72.
19. Derek S. Hyra, "Conceptualizing the New Urban Renewal: Comparing the Past to the Present," *Urban Affairs Review* 48, no. 4 (2012): 505.

Hospitals and other parts of the U.S. health care sector participate in these efforts to revalorize devalued landscapes. This is especially visible in the redevelopment of urban military areas, where, in spite of remediation requirements, property redevelopment promises high returns and reduced risk to developers. St. Anthony Central Hospital in Denver, Colorado, for example, took advantage of a land deal to relocate the facility to a land parcel formerly part of the Denver Federal Center and its World War II–era military ordnance testing range. This brownfield move enabled the hospital to turn over its previous location for a profit. The Denver Urban Renewal Authority has redeveloped the former 18.85-acre St. Anthony campus in the West Colfax neighborhood, including a nearly $40 million TIF-financed rehabilitation of a 44,000-square-foot building that features retail and restaurant space as well as market-rate townhomes.[20] With no shortage of brownfields from military activity along Colorado's Front Range, the Denver suburb of northwest Aurora converted the Fitzsimons Army Medical Center into the 227-acre Anschutz Medical Campus for the University of Colorado and the University of Colorado Hospital.[21] Since the base closed, the Fitzsimons area has become one of the largest medical redevelopment projects in the United States, requiring remediation of three military landfills that reportedly comprise the largest landfill remediation effort in the state of Colorado.[22] A combined Anschutz

20. DURA Renew Denver, "St. Anthony Block 3," accessed November 7, 2022, https://renewdenver.org/projects/st-anthony-block-3/; Ed Sealover, "EFG Brownfield Buying Centura's Old St. Anthony Hospital Site," *Denver Business Journal,* November 11, 2011, https://www.bizjournals.com/denver/news/2011/11/10/denver-buyer-found-for-old-st-as.html.

21. U.S. Department of Defense, "Fitzsimons Army Medical Center, Colorado Redevelopment Profile," October 2020, https://oldcc.gov/project/fitzsimons-army-medical-center-colorado-redevelopment-profile.

22. Matrix, "Fitzsimons (Sand Creek) Parkway and Landfill Remediation," accessed November 7, 2022, https://www.matrixdesign-group.com/fitzsimons-sand-creek-parkway-landfill-remediation; "Notice of Record of Decision for the Disposal and Reuse of the Former Fitzsimons

Medical Campus and Fitzsimons Life Science District are undergoing an over $4 billion transformation into a multizone educational, research, and clinical national center. Hospitals take advantage of brownfield strategies in their real estate pursuits; this raises questions about public process, accountability, and governance of remediation. Such remediation efforts may entail less stringent environmental cleanup standards at the sites where medical services will be provided.

Hospital rehabilitations and expansions also claim immense resources under the auspices of improving the environment, ameliorating urban poverty, and lifting property values, even as they continue to play a role in perpetuating uneven geographies of health and property value in the regional economy. Examining the policy environment and practice of this medical brownfield frontier through the policy arena known as Eds and Meds further delineates the toxic, extractive, and racist property system in which biomedical land developers participate and profit. Eds and Meds development policies seek to remedy postindustrial blight and contamination and foster urban growth tied to research university medical centers and teaching hospitals, which are perceived as powerful economic engines. The policy framework stems from decades-long discussions of "anchor institutions" as a critical component of inner-city revitalization strategies. The basic idea is that benefits from anchor-based economic development will eventually trickle down to inner-city residents in the form of jobs, access to services, and neighborhood amenities.[23] Advocates insist that these institutions have the capacity to create centers of innovation and learning with a large stake and important presence in cities and their surrounding communities.

Army Medical Center," 63 F.R. 16770, *Federal Register* 63, no. 65 (1998), https://www.govinfo.gov/app/details/FR-1998-04-06/98-8854.

23. Robert Mark Silverman, Jade Lewis, and Kelly L. Patterson, "William Worthy's Concept of 'Institutional Rape' Revisited: Anchor Institutions and Residential Displacement in Buffalo, N.Y.," *Humanity and Society* 38, no. 2 (2014): 163.

Accordingly, they are job generators with multilevel employment possibilities; they attract businesses, highly skilled individuals, and spin-off ventures; and they consume sizable amounts of land and are unlikely to relocate.[24] Research on Eds and Meds highlights the contributions hospitals specifically make to cities in terms of expenditures, employment, and real estate development, especially their investments in facilities and specialized technology. Some hospitals have large land holdings located in central cities; others serve as a focal point of ancillary health care businesses, including physicians and medical specialists. These institutions are increasingly part of medical campuses that include facilities dedicated to medical education, biomedical research, long-term care, and outpatient care.

Thus, "Meds" usually refers to teaching-intensive, high-income hospitals and some specialty hospitals—those powerful and resource-rich acute care facilities that are likely to spend money on community economic development and promote health missions tied to generating economic returns on land redevelopment. These elite Meds, which are predominantly nonprofit institutions exempt from federal, state, and local taxes, take center stage in urban governance efforts to offset the costs of city services and to stimulate local growth. Because the health care sector has been one of the few consistent economic growth areas in U.S. cities through the late twentieth and early twenty-first centuries, city officials see elite hospitals or systems as generators of new monies with spillover effects.[25] Institutions like the Cleveland Clinic, University of Alabama Hospital, University of Pittsburgh Medical Center, and other university-affiliated hospitals offer export-based industry status: they provide clinical training for medical students and health care professionals, and physicians on staff frequently are experts in

24. Henry Louis Taylor Jr. and Gavin Luter, "Anchor Institutions: An Interpretive Review Essay," Anchor Institution Task Force, 2013, https://community-wealth.org/content/anchor-institutions-interpretive-review-essay, 8.

25. McKee, "Health-Care Policy," 3.

their field with access to the most advanced equipment.[26] By attracting in-migration and developing human capital, such hospitals are hailed for growing entrepreneurship and prioritizing diverse local suppliers.[27] City officials especially look to Meds' campus investments to increase land values. Their dominant policy approach has been to position biomedical institutions as land developers by using municipal authority to assemble land parcels for campus expansions and by engaging in public–private or public–public partnerships that target neighborhood development.[28] When institutional improvements drive up neighboring land values, the city's increased revenues help compensate for the property tax exemptions that the institutions enjoy.[29] Moreover, hospital development is perceived to be a place-making activity capable of maximizing welfare and distributional equity, reducing intrametro disparities, and offering formal strategies of upward mobility in employment like skills attainment and credentialing for inner-city communities. Moral arguments surround Eds and Meds policy, including social responsibility and a pedagogic duty to provide models of responsible citizenship and good neighborliness—civic virtues that supposedly can be mobilized to embed capital accumulation in public service.[30] Such appeals are used to justify the tax exemptions that these institutions enjoy.

This policy framework, however, implants a nonprofit medical complex in American cities, particularly those in financial distress and near–municipal bankruptcy conditions, by offering tax breaks

26. McKee, "Health-Care Policy," 3; Marla Nelson, "Are Hospitals an Export Industry? Empirical Evidence from Five Lagging Regions," *Economic Development Quarterly* 23, no. 3 (2009): 248.

27. Howard K. Koh, Amy Bantham, Alan C. Geller, et al., "Anchor Institutions: Best Practices to Address Social Needs and Social Determinants of Health," *American Journal of Public Health* 110, no. 3 (2020): 311.

28. Carolyn Adams, "The Meds and Eds in Urban Economic Development," *Journal of Urban Affairs* 25, no. 5 (2003): 578.

29. Adams, "Meds and Eds," 578.

30. Taylor and Luter, "Anchor Institutions," 13.

in exchange for trickle-down benefits. Participating institutions are able to exploit public subsidies and devalued land; they implement predatory forms of financial extraction using the colonial rhetoric of educational mission and nonprofit charity work. Eds and Meds create and exploit medical brownfields that locally manifest in some of the worst disease rates and racialized health disparities in the United States at the very sites of top national and renowned hospital care. This colonial process encourages and organizes land grabs that are based on discourses of blight and waste-ability, imposes fiscal eminent domain that channels resources to development authorities and their territorial projects, and claims to offset the corrosive effects of this brownfield frontier on surrounding residents through local benefits and sustainability initiatives. A poignant example, medical administration and care in Camden, New Jersey, demonstrates the institutionalization of racial inequity in ways that reveal how some Meds projects intensify geographies of waste and race, stripping assets with devastating effects on local residents.[31] After the collapse of its manufacturing base and decades of white flight and disinvestment, Camden has turned to large-scale waste processing—a regional sewage treatment plant, open-air sewage sludge composting facility, trash-to-steam incinerator, power-cogeneration facility, coke transfer station, chemical companies, cement-grinding plants, and more—as the means to reverse industrial decline within a deeply racialized region. The presence of these toxic industries, combined with poverty and violent crime, all have contributed to a dire public health problem in Camden, where the city's residents are majority Black and Latinx. In the same area of this proliferating waste industry and humanitarian crisis, Camden currently hosts a growing nonprofit medical complex that facilitates developmentalist nongovernmental organization interventions to help poor people who have inadequate health care. Politicians have pushed

---

31. Diane Sicotte, *From Workshop to Waste Magnet: Environmental Inequality in the Philadelphia Region* (Newark, N.J.: Rutgers University Press, 2016).

an Eds and Meds approach to land redevelopment, with higher education and health care nonprofits as anchor institutions for the city's "rebirth," along with the state's designation of Camden as a growth zone that offers major tax breaks.[32]

On one end of the spectrum, Camden has innovated a data-based approach to decreasing exorbitant health care spending on the medically indigent. This strategy, known as "medical hot spotting," entails sharing medical metadata across hospitals, jails, and schools; it uses GIS technologies to locate and target "high utilizers" of intensive, uncompensated outpatient care, for the purposes of motivating them to do better self-care and cost the system less.[33] Such "care" tries to integrate people within the surveillance of poverty. This has reportedly included job training for residents in medical data entry to support a medical intelligence industry that intensifies the division of labor of managing the poor. Medical hot spotting also remains wedded to a biomedical model of intervention that does not address Camden's environmental health conditions, where long-standing environmental justice activism has fought widespread toxicity and hazards that attenuate quality of life, including some of the highest asthma rates in the country.[34] Camden has attracted high-end hospitals, such as the research facility and teaching-oriented Cooper University Hospital, that operate with little reference to the surrounding poverty and environmental health inequities experienced by Camden residents. The affluence of this elite nonprofit institution and other trophy companies purportedly

32. U.S. EPA, "Camden, New Jersey Uses Green Infrastructure to Manage Stormwater," accessed November 7, 2022, https://www.epa.gov/arc-x/camden-new-jersey-uses-green-infrastructure-manage-stormwater.

33. Nadine Ehlers and Shiloh Krupar, *Deadly Biocultures: The Ethics of Life-making* (Minneapolis: University of Minnesota Press), 46–68.

34. New Jersey Department of Health, "Camden County Public Health Profile Report: Asthma Hospitalizations and Emergency Department Visits, 2020," data updated February 10, 2022, https://www-doh.state.nj.us/doh-shad/community/highlight/profile/NJASTHMAHOSP.countyAAR/GeoCnty/4.html.

trickles down to the local population, yet the tax exemptions that drew them to Camden facilitate billions in private profits and lost property taxes, thus stripping the city of its tax base.[35] Their infrastructural demands, security theater, and philanthropic support for local amenities like parks and heritage district revivals perpetuate and obscure violence within the urban community.

The land development strategies of the Cleveland Clinic in Cleveland, Ohio, underscore how nonprofit hospital tax exemptions may intensify legacies of Jim Crow segregation. The nonprofit academic medical center's unrelenting expansion of operations—what local African American residents have characterized as "the plantation"—thrives on the surrounding neighborhoods' dereliction and abandonment.[36] The main campus occupies an ever-expanding seventeen-block stretch of land, with smooth roads, paved bike lanes, and glassy white buildings connected by skyways. The campus has its own private police force, hosts a high-end InterContinental Hotel, and offers a variety of amenities akin to an airport terminal or resort, with live music, shopping, and a farmers market. The second biggest employer in Ohio (just behind Walmart), pride of Cleveland, and one of the most prestigious hospitals in the world, the Cleveland Clinic's treatment of the land and surrounding neighborhoods as a special medical district and development platform has led to starkly uneven health care disparities. One of the best-known global brands in health care buttresses local conditions of medical apartheid. The surrounding neighborhood of Fairfax has an infant mortality rate nearly three times the national average; more than one third of residents in the census tract surrounding the clinic have diabetes; and the predominantly African American population experiences

35. Nancy Solomon and Jeff Pillets, "How Companies and Allies of One Powerful Democrat Got $1.1 Billion in Tax Breaks," *ProPublica,* May 1, 2019, https://www.propublica.org/article/george-norcross-democratic-donor-tax-breaks.

36. Dan Diamond, "How the Cleveland Clinic Grows Healthier While Its Neighbors Stay Sick," *Politico,* July 17, 2017, https://www.politico.com/interactives/2017/obamacare-cleveland-clinic-non-profit-hospital-taxes/.

higher rates of cancer, chronic kidney disease, and coronary heart disease.[37] While wealthy international patients receive heart transplants at the clinic, local people do not go there for an emergency; in fact, the hospital has been sued for not providing enough emergency care. Like many high-end hospitals, attracting wealthy patients and expanding operations to global cities such as London, Toronto, and Abu Dhabi take precedence over serving poor patients for Medicaid rates or receiving the fractional payouts and charity write-offs for treating the uninsured.

As a tax-exempt organization, the Cleveland Clinic saves tens of millions in annual property taxes from its billion-dollar property value, with only a loosely defined commitment to reinvest in the local community. The clinic claims that it is in fact improving the surrounding area, which is beset with vacant lots, abandoned structures, and bail-bond outfits, and that its world-renowned physicians and well-paying jobs lift up the community. Yet in a grotesque extension of urban renewal's draining of wealth from inner-city areas through investments in white suburbs and highways, the institution has pursued an over $300 million project called the Opportunity Corridor. Construction of this three-mile highway requires ripping up streets and tearing down residential and commercial buildings, ultimately to expedite shuttling staff and patients to the hospital's sea of parking garages from Interstate 490.[38] The boulevard construction vacuums up what could have been the clinic's property taxes and local investments in schools and city services: providing out-of-hospital care and social support, acculturating local workers successfully in clinic jobs, monitoring neighborhood health, and engaging in land remediation to address lead exposure are equally as important as treating heart attacks.[39] The Cleveland Clinic reveals

37. Diamond, "How the Cleveland Clinic."

38. Steven Litt, "Opportunity Corridor Is Back on Track for 2021 Completion after Delay Caused by Taxpayer Lawsuit," *Cleveland.com*, February 14, 2018, https://www.cleveland.com/architecture/2018/02/opportunity_corridor_on_track.html.

39. Cleveland Clinic does support the nearby Langston Hughes Community Health and Education Center.

the way that medical brownfields service extraterritorial enterprise zones that perpetuate financial, infrastructural, and medical redlining across generations and transnational space. As home foreclosures continue to unfold, with Cleveland a ground zero for the 2008 subprime mortgage crisis and its predatory lending targeted at Black citizens, the racist tautology of home repossession as dispossession has provided the terrain for the clinic's most ambitious land grabs yet. Clinic master plans reenvision the surrounding East Cleveland neighborhoods as a blank slate for a continuous "green spine" campus park, revealing the colonial operations of a green brownfield frontier and renewed rounds of *redlining as greenlining.* The ongoing racial violence of the Covid-19 pandemic has given the clinic further rationale for land grabs, supporting a humanitarian spectacle that obscures its parasitical relationship to place. The clinic is currently developing an over $500 million "innovation district" that will feature world-class research institutes devoted to Covid-19 and other global pathogens. It is to be placed on land comprising the historically Black neighborhood of Hough, which has been devastated by Covid—further compounding the previous waves of foreclosure and hospital land seizures after racial uprisings.[40]

Johns Hopkins University (JHU) has been the largest landholder and biggest builder in Baltimore; it has even formed its own full-service real estate development subsidiary, which offers a range of expertise in land planning, financing, construction, and property management for tenants of its medical center.[41] The Johns Hopkins Health System has unveiled plans for a $400 million, twelve-story research tower on its East Baltimore main campus,

40. More than $200 million in state money will support the new building and job creation tax credits, buoying the partnership between the Cleveland Clinic, University Hospitals, MetroHealth, Case Western Reserve University, and Cleveland State University.

41. Charles Belfoure, "$1 Billion in Projects for Johns Hopkins in Baltimore," *New York Times*, February 6, 2000, https://www.nytimes.com/2000/02/06/realestate/1-billion-in-projects-for-johns-hopkins-in-baltimore.html.

which will solidify its status as a global medical research hub.[42] Constituting an even larger part of JHU's footprint in Baltimore is the East Baltimore Development Inc.'s massive eighty-eight-acre territory, which seeks to leverage its proximity to the Hopkins Homewood campus and provide millions of square feet in life sciences research and office space, in addition to mixed-income housing, schools, parks, and retail.[43] After years of delays and setbacks, the project has aggressively torn down approximately two thousand of the surrounding neighborhood rowhouses and relocated over seven hundred families. What was once the thriving blue-collar Black neighborhood known as Middle East has been rebranded Eager Park. In spite of East Baltimore Development's careful language and emphasis on Black citizens returning to a renewed neighborhood, the project bears a striking similarity to previous JHU-led property occupation and expansion, including a fifty-nine-acre urban renewal project that displaced more than a thousand families in the 1950s.[44] The zoning maps delineate a medical brownfield frontier wherein every census block has been placed in the bottom categories of "stressed" and in need of "comprehensive housing market interventions . . . including site

42. Ed Gunts, "Johns Hopkins Health System Unveils Plans for $400 Million, 12-Story Research Tower," *Baltimore Fishbowl,* November 7, 2019, https://baltimorefishbowl.com/stories/johns-hopkins-health-system-unveils-plans-for-400-million-12-story-research-tower/.

43. Jason Richardson, Bruce Mitchell, and Juan Franco of National Community Reinvestment Coalition, "Shifting Neighborhoods: Gentrification and Cultural Displacement in American Cities," March 19, 2019, https://ncrc.org/gentrification/; Lawrence T. Brown, *The Black Butterfly: The Harmful Politics of Race and Space in America* (Baltimore, Md.: Johns Hopkins University Press, 2021).

44. Steve Hendrix, "Johns Hopkins Hospital Inspires Mistrust and Fear in Parts of East Baltimore," *Washington Post,* February 2, 2017, https://www.washingtonpost.com/local/johns-hopkins-hospital-inspires-mistrust-and-fear-in-parts-of-east-baltimore/2017/01/25/a4f402c2-bbf3-11e6-91ee-1adddfe36cbe_story.html; Siddhartha Mitter, "Gentrify or Die? Inside a University's Controversial Plan for Baltimore," *Guardian,* April 18, 2018, https://www.theguardian.com/cities/2018/apr/18/gentrify-or-die-inside-a-universitys-controversial-plan-for-baltimore.

assembly, tax increment financing, and concentrated demolitions to create potential for greater public safety and new green amenities."[45] Residents and activists have fought for fair compensation and relocation terms, as well as to ensure demolitions are conducted safely, without stirring up massive contaminants. Thus far the redevelopment zone features housing exclusively for graduate students, a new public school with very few spots for local children, renovated rowhouses and a townhome complex that JHU heavily subsidizes for its employees, and a Marriott Residence Inn facing a park on a block where forty rowhouses once stood.

In a move indicative of the national prioritizing of citadels of acute care against urban unrest, the privately held, multibillion-dollar operation of JHU simultaneously seeks the authority to establish its own armed police force to secure its Baltimore urban campus and hospital, as well as its domestic and global facilities. After the uprisings in response to the death of Freddie Gray in police custody in 2015, JHU has spent more than half a million dollars lobbying for expanded policing powers that increase the risk of racial profiling and brutality for students, employees, and members of the surrounding community, although it suspended the effort momentarily in 2020 during the global Black Lives Matter protests and civil uprisings.[46] Such private police forces across the

45. Mittel, "Gentrify or Die?," drawing on Dax-Devlon Ross, "The Great East Baltimore Raze-and-Rebuild," *Next City,* July 29, 2013, https://nextcity.org/features/the-great-east-baltimore-raze-and-rebuild; Baltimore Department of Planning, "Description of Housing Market Typology Map," accessed November 7, 2022, https://planning.baltimorecity.gov/housing-market-typology/descriptions-housing-market-typology-map; Sara Safransky, "Rethinking Land Struggle in the Postindustrial City," *Antipode* 49, no. 4 (2017): 1079–100.

46. Lillian Reed and Tim Prudente, "Johns Hopkins University to Move Forward with Private Police Force," *Baltimore Sun,* July 27, 2021, https://www.baltimoresun.com/education/bs-md-hopkins-public-safety-20210727-20210727-djzghhbaebczpi52yaudzfhs5q-story.html. JHU students, faculty, and community residents engaged in a month-long sit-in at the university's main administration that led to numerous arrests.

country receive little public oversight or scrutiny, yet their officers carry weapons and often operate with full police power on campus and across adjacent city blocks.[47] JHU contends that these resources are necessary to safeguard its educational mission and partnerships with the city. The situation reflects the decades-long parallel public policy track of "investing in cutting-edge, high-tech solutions and an emergency medicine system that has been a poor fit for the general health of many Americans, especially the poor and uninsured who lack adequate facilities and basic care in their communities" while also investing in police forces and systems of incarceration that disproportionately harm BIPOC communities and exacerbate the convergent American health epidemics of racism and gun violence.[48] Nic John Ramos explains that cities have prioritized resources for publicly funded emergency medical response, prisons, police, and fire departments while defunding public hospitals, clinics, and health education programs. This has essentially subsidized state-of-the-art facilities like JHU for privately insured Americans and global consumers; these facilities offer costly acute care and emergency services, especially for rare and singular diseases or for end-of-life care, instead of developing capacities for low-cost preventive health care to support health equity and guide reparative justice in everyday life and death.[49] The extreme life-threatening health disparities of Baltimore residents exemplify the damaging effects of this discriminatory convergence of health and urban policy. Indeed, the *Washington Post* reports

47. David Armstrong, "The Startling Reach and Disparate Impact of Cleveland Clinic's Private Police Force," *ProPublica,* September 28, 2020, https://www.propublica.org/article/what-trump-and-biden-should-debate-at-the-cleveland-clinic-why-the-hospitals-private-police-mostly-arrest-black-people.

48. Nic John Ramos, "Solving Our Urban Crisis Involves Addressing Hospitals in Addition to Policing," *Washington Post,* June 1, 2020, https://www.washingtonpost.com/outlook/2020/06/01/solving-our-urban-crisis-involves-addressing-hospitals-addition-policing/.

49. Ramos, "Solving Our Urban Crisis."

that in a city with one of the country's premier health institutions, average life expectancy in numerous Baltimore neighborhoods is lower than that of economically collapsed countries in colonial war zones, with eight ranking lower than Syria. If the life expectancy of residents of the affluent neighborhood of Baltimore's Roland Park is similar to Japan's, then that of residents of the downtown/Seton Hill area is closer to Yemen's.[50]

These city cases reveal tautologies of racial violence. U.S. urban policies have driven hospitals toward property-oriented growth, with racially oppressive responses to urban unrest. U.S. health policies have supported a model of private health care citadels with emergency services in the context of general medical scarcity for poor and uninsured people. The property-based orientation of Eds and Meds boosterism enacts a brownfield frontier imagination that facilitates colonial land grabs in the name of urban revitalization, sustainability initiatives, local place making, and other extensions of the discourse of blight. It fails to consider how anchor institutions were born from land theft, public subsidies, and, in the case of advanced acute care and premier hospitals, biopiracy and the medical abuse of nonwhite and vulnerable subjects.[51] The historical grave robbing of Black bodies and the stealing of Henrietta Lack's cancer cells for medical research supported the very rise of Johns Hopkins as a renowned research university that today receives more federal research funding than any other.[52]

50. Christopher Ingraham, "14 Baltimore Neighborhoods Have Lower Life Expectancies than North Korea," *Washington Post*, April 30, 2015, https://www.washingtonpost.com/news/wonk/wp/2015/04/30/baltimores-poorest-residents-die-20-years-earlier-than-its-richest/.

51. Harriet A. Washington, *Medical Apartheid: The Dark History of Medical Experimentation on Black Americans from Colonial Times to the Present* (New York: Anchor, 2008).

52. Nick Anderson, Lauren Lumpkin, and Susan Svrluga, "Johns Hopkins, Benefactor of Namesake Hospital and University, Was an Enslaver," *Washington Post*, December 9, 2020, https://www.washingtonpost.com/local/education/johns-hopkins-slavery/2020/12/09/cf0744f6-3a30-11eb-98c4-25dc9f4987e8_story.html.

Such cases demonstrate some of the ways that medical brown-fields reterritorialize governance in the austerity state. They create a fiscal environment for complex quasi-public mechanisms, territorial policing, and other powers that facilitate local large-scale land redevelopments, skirting neoliberal retrenchment of federal assistance and often bypassing legislative hurdles, electoral politics, and long-established constitutional limits on debt.[53] This third sector of the U.S. economy, which combines marketplace and governance and which operates outside the boundaries of formal government, can in part be traced back to nonprofit public benefit corporations and municipal improvement authorities advanced by U.S. presidents Hoover and Roosevelt since the 1930s as a way to build public works without bankrupting municipal treasuries. Instead of using taxes and direct payment to pay for projects, these quasi-public development authorities split from electoral politics to redevelop land and pay for projects by borrowing against future revenues.[54] More recently, the neoliberal era has seen a profusion of special-purpose authorities, commissions, and partnerships that make it easier to borrow money without that debt counting as part of a city's total indebtedness, thus circumventing debt limits as well as the reporting requirements of government departments. For example, a twenty-year economic development initiative, Destination Medical Center, authorizes public investments and public governance structure to help support the Mayo Clinic's continual growth via a $5.6 billion plan to convert Rochester, Minnesota, into a global medical destination center. The Destination Medical Center master plan seeks to transform Rochester's urban center and waterfront into six subdistricts to serve as an extension of the Mayo Clinic.

---

53. These political and financial mechanisms are much older than the neoliberal era. See Albert M. Spragia, *Debt Wish: Entrepreneurial Cities, U.S. Federalism, and Economic Development* (Pittsburgh, Pa.: University of Pittsburgh Press, 1996).

54. Carolyn Adams, "Urban Governance and the Control of Infrastructure," *Public Works Management and Policy* 11, no. 3 (2007): 164–65.

The plan remasters Rochester in the Mayo Clinic's image, complete with a rebranded downtown and a slogan, "The Heart of the City," referring to Mayo's expertise in cardiology and heart surgery.[55]

With the proliferation of municipal regimes that actively make landscapes amenable to quick excavation of value, redevelopment authorities function as debt machines without voter approval. These regimes do not have to consult the electorate over spending and borrowing; they can raise revenue through user fees, grants, and bond issuances on the capital markets.[56] Advocates of market discipline aver that self-supporting enterprise funds and public authorities are possible and desirable, but in actuality, they are not free from the broader political economy and can have negative effects within racialized urban regions, as the examples above have considered. Establishing development authorities diverts city revenues to pursue pro-growth development, often resulting in property speculation and public giveaways that guide the "place and pace of the speculative activity."[57] Once a redevelopment project is created, all property tax increment directly channels to the agency in charge, when such funds could have been used to keep open libraries, staff emergency rooms, and support other urgently needed services. Redevelopment authorities perform eminent domain in not only a territorial sense but also a fiscal one. Such medical brownfields perform what Clyde Woods calls "trap economics": they strip local assets and transfer wealth.[58]

Discourses surrounding hospitals as urban anchors and growth machines solicit mass support by appeals to trickle-down bene-

55. Destination Medical Center, "Development Plan, Vol. 1—Executive Summary and Phase I Strategies," April 23, 2015, https://dmc.mn/wp-content/plugins/pdf-viewer-for-wordpress/web/viewer.php?file=/wp-content/uploads/2018/07/Executive-Summary.pdf.

56. Weber, "Extracting Value," 531; Adams, "Urban Governance," 165.

57. Weber, "Extracting Value," 537.

58. Clyde Woods, "Les Misérables of New Orleans: Trap Economics and the Asset Stripping Blues, Part 1," *American Quarterly* 61, no. 3 (2009): 769–96.

fits. Even as grassroots groups demand concessions and local governments organize community development agreements with job training, educational investments, low-income housing, or other amenities, the trickle-down model facilitates a territorial trap—that is, gentrification processes displace inner-city residents, exacerbating tensions between job creation and property value increases, as well as diminishing municipal capacity to generate revenue for both operating budgets and capital budgets. TIFs, for instance, mount property tax losses for investments at large because money stays in that particular submunicipal territory, foisting the property tax burden for public provisions onto the remaining taxable property owners. Eds and Meds development projects concentrate tax-exempt properties and thus weaken the municipal tax base substantially, adding stress to the delivery of social welfare programs and public services.

Furthermore, the consumer framing of such zones obscures who ultimately pays for the infrastructure and other benefits—as well as the costs, such as inadequately funded maintenance or congestion—that receipt of services imposes on others. Anchor institutions are heavily subsidized by public expenditures and other government resources that form the social safety net in inner-city neighborhoods, including not only brownfield remediation but also housing, parks, grocery stores, and recreational facilities.[59] As land developers, elite nonprofit hospitals prosper in low-revenue municipal environments. A pro-growth rhetoric of place making shrouds the exclusionary practices and fiscal appropriation orchestrated by development authorities that operate outside of democratic process. Despite efforts to retain locally specific obligations, whether related to aesthetics, environmental sustainability, contracting prices, job creation, or diversity, development authorities use highly opaque financial instruments built around idiosyncratic investments and

59. Silverman, Lewis, and Patterson, "William Worthy's Concept," 163–64.

specialized information that can result in pay-to-play scenarios and investment schemes that leave cities encumbered by high-interest debt on usurious terms.[60]

The tax exemption status of a mounting nonprofit philanthro-capitalist medical complex creates an environment where medical brownfields flourish and perpetuate urban blight. Nonprofit hospitals enjoy multiple public subsidies through Medicare and Medicaid, public and private insurance programs, and tax-exempt status. Historically, most hospitals in the United States have been recognized as charitable organizations excepted from taxes under section 501(c)(3) of the U.S. tax code. In exchange, the IRS requires that nonprofit hospitals provide a significant amount of care for the poor, also known as charity care. After Medicare and Medicaid were established in 1965, the hospital industry claimed that there would no longer be enough demand for charity care to fulfill the IRS's tax exemption standard (because Americans would supposedly be covered by one of the two programs or by private health insurance); the industry pushed for a more flexible exemption standard that became known as the "community benefit" standard.[61] While charity care remains a key component, the historical shift indicates the changing vision of civic leaders and legislators toward hospitals and academic medical centers. Beyond simply providing direct patient care, the mission of hospitals could expand to encompass health promotion, poverty relief, education, and a wide range of activities deemed beneficial to the community.[62] The ambiguity of community benefits has allowed many hospitals to include a bewildering array

60. Weber, "Selling City Futures"; Adams, "Urban Governance," 171.

61. John Carreyrou and Barbara Martinez, "Nonprofit Hospitals, Once for the Poor, Strike It Rich," *Wall Street Journal,* April 4, 2008, https://www.wsj.com/articles/SB120726201815287955. The IRS adopted the community benefit standard in 1969.

62. Andrew T. Simpson, "'We Will Gladly Join You in Partnership in Harrisburg or We Will See You in Court': The Growth of Large Not-for-Profits and Consequences of the 'Eds and Meds' Renaissance in the New Pittsburgh," *Journal of Urban History* 42, no. 2 (2016): 308.

of expenses in their accounting to the IRS, including unpaid patient bills and tallies of the difference between the list prices of treatment they provide and what they are paid by Medicaid and Medicare.[63] Contributing to debates about not-for-profit fiscal responsibility, many elite nonprofit hospitals spend significantly less on charity care than the tax breaks they receive. Some Eds and Meds institutions make payments in lieu of taxes, known as PILOTs, to partially offset the foregone property tax revenue. However, this kind of flat fee hardly compensates for the lost revenue or broader costs of providing infrastructure and services, which are shifted to local residents and increase their relative tax burden.[64] As a result, section 501(r) was added to the IRS tax code as part of the Affordable Care Act to further delineate what counts toward tax-exempt status.[65]

Many poverty alleviation programs and career ladder programs are financed with "demonstration" funding and philanthropic contributions in place of public sector investments.[66] Within the hospital sector, policies to engage the poor in employment opportunities exhort people to earn their way out of poverty, but without providing the work-based learning models or mentoring needed to advance along skill and pay tracks. The nonprofitization of federal urban policy has devolved federal funding and decentralized community development policy to the local level, relegating local development to nonprofit networks led by foundations and anchor

63. Carreyrou and Martinez, "Nonprofit Hospitals."

64. Michael A. Pagano, "Financing Infrastructure in the 21st Century City," *Public Works Management and Policy* 13, no. 1 (2008): 29–30. PILOTs started as early as the 1960s.

65. U.S. Internal Revenue Service, "Requirements for 501(c)(3) Hospitals Under the Affordable Care Act—Section 501(r)," last reviewed July 15, 2022, https://www.irs.gov/charities-non-profits/charitable-organizations/requirements-for-501c3-hospitals-under-the-affordable-care-act-section-501r.

66. Marla Nelson and Laura Wolf-Powers, "Chains and Ladders: Exploring the Opportunities for Workforce Development and Poverty Reduction in the Hospital Sector," *Economic Development Quarterly* 24, no. 1 (2010): 42.

institutions. The withdrawal of federal resources designed to assist residents who have been negatively affected by urban redevelopment has meant that cities must rely on philanthropic contributions to support any social safety net, and urban residents in need of public services must negotiate a complex web of organizations engaged in urban revitalization.[67] Pro-growth Eds and Meds urban policies offer dubious improvements to the actual health care quality and wellness of neighboring residents and local workers.[68] As employers, these institutions notoriously set the nonprofessional wage ceiling in cities, with their reliance on tiers of lower-waged workers, including technicians, nurse's aides, custodians, and food service workers.[69] Elite medical campuses that attract nonresidents seeking state-of-the-art medical treatments may actually contribute to reducing access to general health services for local indigent populations.[70] Health care markets harm low-income people when competition among medical facilities erodes the cross-subsidies that have financed access to care.

Undoubtedly many hospitals serve as integral components of the social safety net by filling in roles as primary providers of publicly subsidized health care. Numerous nonprofit institutions support local government provision of public goods and have organized a variety of public assets or concessions, including affordable housing, improvements to schools and community facilities, local employment, returning-citizen recruitment, job training, and minority procurement. The Greater University Circle Initiative, for example, a

67. Silverman, Lewis, and Patterson, "William Worthy's Concept," 161.

68. Timothy J. Bartik and George Erickcek, "The Local Economic Impact of 'Eds and Meds': How Policies to Expand Universities and Hospitals Affect Metropolitan Economies," *Brookings,* December 10, 2008, https://www.brookings.edu/research/the-local-economic-impact-of-eds-meds-how-policies-to-expand-universities-and-hospitals-affect-metropolitan-economies/, 14.

69. Baldwin, *In the Shadow,* 48.

70. Silverman, Lewis, and Patterson, "William Worthy's Concept," 163; Nelson, "Are Hospitals an Export Industry?"

partnership between the Cleveland Foundation and local advocates with Case Western Reserve University, University Hospitals, and the Cleveland Clinic, has sought to boost income and opportunities for residents of the seven low-income neighborhoods surrounding them by collaborating on transportation infrastructure, pooling purchasing power, and channeling business to local, employee-owned cooperatives.[71] In other cases, teaching hospitals have organized programs that place medical students in local high schools to promote health, or to facilitate communication among local leaders of faith, schools, neighborhood organizations, and clinics. Such contributions emanate from hard-fought local struggles and decades of activism; they are the fruit of long-term public demands for community benefit agreements to support inner-city residents affected by the expansion of anchors.

Even as cities face financial conditions that make it difficult to justify public investments that are not fiscally productive, some elected officials and local states have pressured hospitals and health systems into providing more community support, vehemently criticizing the disparity between the charity care and benefits offered by hospitals compared to their tax exemptions and CEO incomes. This is in part due to the changing nonprofit model, which has come to resemble that of for-profits under conditions of vigorous price competition.[72] A business model mimicking for-profit strategies has incentivized the creation of not-for-profit corporate structures and integrated academic health systems, with huge increases in

71. Koh et al., "Anchor Institutions," 313. The antagonistic relationship between East Cleveland neighborhoods and the development citadel of University Circle spans decades. See J. Mark Souther, "Acropolis of the Middle-West: Decay, Renewal, and Boosterism in Cleveland's University Circle," *Journal of Planning History* 10, no. 1 (2011): 30–58.

72. Randall R. Bovbjerg and Jill A. Marsteller, "Health Care Market Competition in Six States: Implications for the Poor," Occasional Paper 17, *Urban Institute,* November 1998, https://www.urban.org/sites/default/files/publication/66621/307916-Health-Care-Market-Competition-in-Six-States. PDF, 2.

recorded earnings and extractive relations with their local places and ecologies. Between 2001 and 2006, the combined net income of the largest nonprofit hospitals jumped nearly eightfold to $4.27 billion, with the Cleveland Clinic leaving the red to run up a net income of $229 million during that period. The nonprofit hospital system Ascension Health had amassed $7.4 billion through that time period.[73] Much of the nonprofit hospital industry's income growth has come from predatory strategies designed to increase revenue, among them prioritizing expensive procedures; greatly inflating list prices for procedures and services; requiring up-front payment; selling patient debt to collection companies; and issuing tax-exempt bonds and investing the proceeds in higher-yielding securities.[74]

This has exacerbated the massive disparities and operational asymmetries between various parts of the health system. Nonprofit hospitals with considerable market power draw in wealthy clients and export services, divisively creating an impoverished peripheral set of charity-oriented nonprofit hospitals that face constant poverty triage, and tax-paying, for-profit inner-city hospitals geared toward stockpiling Medicaid patients. In the rapidly changing health care sector, academic medical center power increases, while other hospitals face extreme austerity measures and closure. A few highly competitive hospital networks have evolved that provide only limited care for the poor, excluding many of the nonprofit and public safety net hospitals that are financially distressed and unable to compete for private patients to stay afloat and offset the cost of subsidizing uncompensated care. In short, biomedical complexes and planned developments in which university teaching hospitals build out life science research facilities, specialty medical facilities, and myriad urban destination features depend on blight in surrounding neighborhoods through their extraction of land and predation on collective fiscal and social capacity. They burden residents with

73. Carreyrou and Martinez, "Nonprofit Hospitals," drawing on a *Wall Street Journal* analysis of data from the American Hospital Directory.
74. Carreyrou and Martinez, "Nonprofit Hospitals."

disproportionate tax loads and subsidies. They dump the fallout from expensive and inaccessible health care in the United States onto other hospitals.

This chapter has examined the domestic frontier of medical brownfields as territorial and fiscal enclaves that extract from the public sector and thrive on blight in various ways. In chapter 3, I turn to medical brownfields in the context of the international joint ventures and global medical entrepôts of elite U.S. hospital systems. The discussion considers how these medical nonprofits further entrench racialized disparities in global health via their transnational extension of specialty services, educative missions, and edifying development aesthetics.

3. Global Medical Entrepôts and U.S. Health Care Inequality

A PROFIT-DRIVEN biomedical model of health fuels the United States' inadequate access to health care and insurance coverage, contributing to the excessive costs of the overall U.S. health care system. This arrangement has facilitated the expansion of urban medical complexes and fueled the growth of the urban health care anchor as a replacement or major supplement to declining manufacturing at the core of urban economies. While a hospital can benefit community development as a major employer and service provider, its very success as an urban economic anchor can exacerbate the systemic cost problems of U.S. health care as a whole.[1] The United States spends the most of any nation by far on its health care system, which focuses on global outreach of acute care for those with the means to afford it as well as emergency care to address domestic poverty crises.[2] With spiraling health care expenditures facilitating the placement of blame on the public sector, the United States has further invested in a corporatized and privatized approach to medicine and public health under the belief that a health market

1. McKee, "Health-Care Policy," 3.
2. Matthew J. Eckelman and Jodi Sherman, "Environmental Impacts of the U.S. Health Care System and Effects on Public Health," *PLoS One* 11, no. 6 (2016): 2.

can best regulate costs and quality.[3] International trade agreements and financial institutions have catalyzed this commercialization of health globally. Capitalizing on the universal desire to improve health, multinational corporations enter other national public health systems to offer privatized care and disseminate technologies, medical goods and services, and costly innovations. The U.S. health care system supports the anchoring of extractive local practices to revenue-seeking overseas joint ventures and global medical entrepôts that promise American intellectual goods, services, and brand names. These activities are promoted through moralizing discourses of global medical progress and educational mission, yet contribute to vastly inequitable divisions between those who benefit from the current system's specialized resource-intensive medical services and those who are subjected to the extractive work and adverse social effects of these biomedical operations.

This chapter scrutinizes the U.S. health care system's entrepreneurial specialty services and medical development complex. This complex features medical centers and hospital networks involved in property-driven development that now seek to establish global clinical research, elite hospitality services, and transnational franchising. The promise of medical technology and expertise enlisted by these globalizing U.S. hospitals conveys a message of deep concern for public health while also supporting the quest for new sources of income and subjects that heed the call for an educative "common good" invested in American training and technology. Their campuses play an important role in the U.S. global health landscape as medical entrepôts of clinical care, research, policy, medical education, and health partnerships. Bolstered by international free trade agreements, these medical centers accumulate capital through parasitical relations with other national health systems. Their competition has ballooned costs and further exposed medical professional ethics and philanthropic claims of civic benevolence to the global

3. Howard Waitzkin, *Medicine and Public Health at the End of Empire* (London: Routledge, 2016), 125.

marketplace.[4] Moreover, by adopting the technocratic discourse of sustainability with its emphasis on administrative, operational, and building-oriented efficiencies, this complex avers environmental responsibility wedded to a transnational development aesthetics of spectacle and luxury. Such efforts advance health colonialism by favoring deregulation, privatization, public sector austerity, and the market-based conversion of user/patient into client/consumer as the means to secure medical quality and health rights. In this geopolitical-economic context, the increased policy emphasis on sustainability in American health care (and global health more generally) compounds the transnational stratification of health; it promotes a technocratic fix in lieu of structural challenges to the political economy of medical services and clinical practices that moors a global medical entrepôt to a domestic medical brownfield within the U.S. empire.

The roots of the modern academic medical center in the United States date back to late nineteenth-century urban development in cities like Baltimore, Boston, and New York City.[5] During the Progressive era, medicine advocated clustering hospitals and medical schools into defined geographic areas. By the 1920s, hosting a medical center with a territorial concentration of services was considered an indispensable civic good. In addition to private donations and philanthropy, medical education received significant government benefits. Federal investment in biomedical research rose fifteenfold, from $87 million in 1947 to $2.05 billion by 1966.[6] As discussed previously, the U.S. federal government offered extensive subsidies to defray indirect costs, such as utilities and mort-

---

4. Waitzkin, *Medicine and Public Health,* 2–4.

5. Simpson, "We Will Gladly Join You," 307. Academic medical centers are uniquely situated in U.S. global health at the intersection of research, clinical care, medical education, global partnerships, and policy.

6. Figures are quoted from Simpson, "We Will Gladly Join You," 307, who draws on Kenneth M. Ludmerer, *Time to Heal: American Medical Education from the Turn of the Century to the Era of Managed Care* (New York: Oxford University Press, 1999), 141–42.

gage payments, which allowed medical schools to grow without putting much of their own capital at risk. Hospitals also derived increasing amounts of revenue from patient care; employer-based health insurance and the passage of Medicare and Medicaid in 1965 guaranteed payment and thus substantially reduced the risk of nonpayment that had previously burdened hospitals during the Depression.[7] With fewer stipulations than federal grant money, revenue from clinical services could be used to fund future service-line expansion projects in high-demand areas like emergency medical services, cardiac care, and oncology, which transformed hospitals into multimillion-dollar-a-year enterprises.[8] According to historian Andrew T. Simpson, these successful not-for-profit hospitals were built using "a range of incentives including access to cheap capital through special bonds, public money to support the creation of the venture capital infrastructure needed to help these organizations diversify into lucrative noncore businesses, and built a regional and national narrative around the triumph of the knowledge economy."[9]

The United States has generally valorized expensive technologies and drugs, as well as invasive procedures and intensive labor arrangements, "to save us when we are at our sickest rather than address nonmedical and public health approaches that prevent the onset of serious disease when we are at our healthiest."[10] Ramos explains that U.S. systemic emphasis on acute care and emergency services stems from decades of public policy in response to the 1960s uprisings—what he describes as the cannibalization of safety net health services. Since the 1980s especially, this has resulted in the "super acute" health system and state-of-the-art facilities for

7. Simpson, "We Will Gladly Join You," 307.
8. Simpson, "We Will Gladly Join You," 308.
9. Simpson, "We Will Gladly Join You," 316–17. See also Andrew T. Simpson, *The Medical Metropolis: Health Care and Economic Transformation in Pittsburgh and Houston* (Philadelphia: University of Pennsylvania Press, 2019).
10. Ramos, "Solving Our Urban Crisis."

privately insured Americans, while the poor and uninsured are treated only through expensive emergency room visits. President Ronald Reagan slashed public health budgets while signing a federal mandate that prohibited hospitals from turning away citizens who need emergency services. Cities have thus prioritized resources for publicly funded emergency medical service systems while de-funding public hospitals and health education projects, essentially redistributing public health resources to subsidize the build-out of cutting-edge, high-tech solutions that massively amplify costs while helping very little to support the general health of Americans, particularly the poor and uninsured who lack basic community resources.[11] The escalating costs of this system are further intensi-fied by the way large nonprofit general hospitals have strategically navigated it, especially their critical role in high-poverty cities. These hospitals often subsidize procedure costs and emergency care charity services with revenues from other procedures. For example, a hospital may bill more for the actual costs of heart surgery or diagnostic imaging in order to use the excess funds to compensate for operations that typically lose money, such as emergency services and charity care for the uninsured.[12]

Under the rationale of cost reduction in medical services, policy changes in the 1990s sought to create price rivalry by generaliz-ing competition among state, social security, and private sectors and by supporting services attractive to managed care plans. In insurance markets, managed care replaced traditional, free-choice-of-provider indemnity coverage. Whereas indemnity plans retro-spectively paid provider-set charges or costs for physical-ordered services from nearly any provider, managed care plans instead used selective contracting to negotiate price and other terms of service

11. This is an encapsulation of several important points of Ramos's argument in "Solving Our Urban Crisis."
12. Devon M. Herrick, "Medical Tourism: Global Competition in Health Care," No. 304, *National Center for Policy Analysis,* November 1, 2007, http://www.ncpathinktank.org/pub/st304, 11.

in advance.[13] Medicare began implementing prospective payments, namely preset reimbursements for services related to diagnosis or procedure for inpatient services. Through selective contracting, managed care plans (in place of individual physicians or patients) negotiated preferable hospital prices. With services and amenities primarily viewed as cost centers, hospitals competed on price by providing services desired by these managed care plans, which were contracting on behalf of large numbers of enrollees and via limited individual subscriber choice.[14] In this provider market, price discounting began to dominate professional and nonprofit determinations of prices and resource allocation in order to compete for health care business and acceptance of fee-for-service Medicare and Medicaid payment limits. By the late 1990s, for-profit managed care organizations entered the public sector to generate profits by keeping costs, especially to pay for services to patients, as low as possible while reaping prepayments funded by public systems. By shifting from national to multinational dimensions, corporations would also export this dominant form of U.S. health care organization to other countries, circumventing national laws to install for-profit investor ownership with prepayment services and other financial rewards from international market extension.[15]

As buyers' demand for less expensive health coverage legitimized and stimulated these market changes, the ostensibly good effects of moving away from free-choice-of-provider indemnity coverage to a managed care structure of risk contracting were attenuated by the negative impacts on access to care for low-income populations. Markets for health care financing and delivery in general affect the extent of enrollment in health coverage, as well as access and quality of care under Medicaid coverage of the uninsured poor,

13. Bovbjerg and Marsteller, "Health Care Market Competition," 1.

14. Robert A. Berenson, Thomas Bodenheimer, and Hoangmai H. Pham, "Specialty-Service Lines: Salvos in the New Medical Arms Race," *Health Affairs* 25 (2006): w337.

15. Waitzkin, *Medicine and Public Health,* 103.

especially charity care provided by hospitals. Competitive price pressures exerted on hospitals prompted hospital budget cutting, along with downsizing, ownership conversion, and consolidation into larger provider entities. Two for-profit chains—Columbia/HCA and Tenet Healthcare—led the charge in consolidating the industry, including purchasing and closing facilities to reduce duplication and excess capacity. Nonprofit systems, such as Adventist Health and Ascension, have also grown and have acquired other hospitals. With doctors, hospitals, insurers, and health plans all functioning as sellers of services that compete on price, quality, and amenities, the U.S. health care system no longer supports independent unaffiliated hospitals and instead favors the amassing of large hospital networks. Moreover, state policies encouraging competition and slashing health care costs have created a "survival of the fittest" model that has caused institutional hardship where competition has been keenest: in the inner cities and metro regions, where urban hospitals bear much of the burden of providing care for the uninsured by virtue of their location and accessibility to large numbers of uninsured patients.[16]

The cost-control imperatives heralded by market-oriented health care reforms have exacerbated conditions of medical scarcity and austerity in urban centers. By using broad discretion over coverage and reimbursement, states have undermined city health care sectors by slashing the number of patients receiving state subsidies and generating more uninsured customers for urban hospitals, cutting reimbursement rates that hospitals receive per patient, and fostering competition between city and suburbs.[17] U.S. health care policy has supported a mode of health care delivery dominated by for-profit managed care companies—and nonprofit systems that operate similarly—undermining the preventive care and quality control that managed care reform in the United States had purportedly valued.[18]

16. Adams, "Meds and Eds," 578, 574.
17. Adams, "Meds and Eds," 574.
18. Waitzkin, *Medicine and Public Health*, 103.

Instead of improving conditions for the poor, market-oriented reforms have deteriorated the public sector safety net, as was made tragically clear when numerous hospitals that pivoted to treat the onslaught of Covid-19 failed because of the dramatic decrease in expensive voluntary procedures at a time of unprecedented need for pandemic-related medical care.[19] Hospital and physician strategies over the last decades have evolved this survival-of-the-fittest model into what some health care commentators call a "medical arms race" among entrepreneurial-oriented medical centers that operate as revenue generators rather than merely as cost centers.[20] Teaching hospitals, for example, have turned to the measure of the marketplace as a dominant standard of value, with the market playing as crucial a role as professional ethics and service.[21] Some of these academic and large nonprofit hospitals have accrued considerable market power by buying up hospitals to establish regional multisite networks and by building expansive urban biomedical complexes, research facilities, physician offices, and even long-term residential care facilities. This has been fueled by the rise of specialty medicine and the proliferation of specialty services. Faced with growing competition for patients, hospitals have in recent decades returned to fee-for-service payments and have adopted strategies dedicated to increasing the flow and filling beds with well-insured patients—a health sector trend that has increased costs and reinforced vertical

19. Howard Waitzkin and Rebecca Jasso-Aguilar, "Empire, Health, and Health Care: Perspectives at the End of Empire as We Have Known It," *Annual Review of Sociology* 41, no. 1 (2015): 276.

20. James C. Robinson and Howard S. Luft, "Competition and the Cost of Hospital Care, 1972 to 1982," *Journal of the American Medical Association* 257, no. 23 (1987): 3241–45; Kelly J. Devers, Linda R. Brewster, and Lawrence P. Casalino, "Changes in Hospital Competitive Strategy: A New Medical Arms Race?" *Health Services Research* 38 (2003): 450.

21. Sidney W. Wolfe, "The Destruction of Medicine by Market Forces: Teaching Acquiescence or Resistance and Change?," *Health Letter* 18, no. 2 (2002): 1–3; Martin Donohoe, "Luxury Primary Care, Academic Medical Centers, and the Erosion of Science and Professional Ethics," *Journal of General Internal Medicine* 19, no. 1 (2004): 92.

schemes focused on specific treatments and diseases rather than universal health coverage and attention to the social and economic dynamics that influence health outcomes.[22]

The ensuing cost-inflating competition partly stems from Reagan-era policy opposition to place-based regulations on medical specialties, such as state-based certificates of need. Such regulations aimed to reduce the duplication of services by requiring health care providers to obtain state approval before offering new or expanded services. However, many states have allowed a proliferation of specialty hospitals and ambulatory care centers that focus exclusively on high-revenue procedures such as cardiac, orthopedic, and outpatient surgery. Such deregulation undermines the place-based welfare function of nonprofit hospitals, instead supporting speculative demand-driven competitive endeavors that purportedly bestow local benefits. Further, this enlarged field of specialty service competition undercuts efforts by individual hospitals to subsidize charity care with high-paying specialty services. By the early 2000s, hospitals were developing and marketing discrete and profitable specialty service lines and engaging in "nonprice competition"—namely retail-oriented, quality dimensions of care and amenities targeted at consumers directly and at physicians who refer patients.[23] This strategy has sought to expand revenue and margins by raising inpatient specialty service volume and adding outpatient centers that can generate additional diagnostic testing and inpatient care.[24] An entreprencurial specialty services and outpatient complex increasingly untethered from charity care and subsidies for emergency response thus dominates American health care provision, escalating already inequitable access to care. Hospitals

22. Jeannie Samuel, review of *Medicine and Public Health at the End of Empire,* by Howard Waitzkin, *Journal of Public Health Policy* 33, no. 2 (2012): 274.

23. Berenson, Bodenheimer, and Pham, "Specialty-Service Lines," w337–38; Devers, Brewster, and Casalino, "Changes in Hospital Competitive Strategy," 447.

24. Devers, Brewster, and Casalino, "Changes in Hospital Competitive Strategy," 458.

continue to add centers for ambulatory surgery, diagnostic testing, and treatment, extending outpatient locations across ever-wider geographic areas in order to increase market presence and referral volume. Teaching hospitals in particular create niche services to attract patients with specific diagnoses to their facilities, aggressively marketing self-designated "centers of excellence" to claim market leadership and establish brand loyalty to attract more patients to their highest-paying services.[25]

Hospitals and physicians are organizing and promoting unique services that are based on specific diseases, organ systems, and populations—heart institutes, orthopedic hospitals, women's clinics, children's services, surgery centers, stroke centers, mental disease specialty clinics, and so forth. Some of these are centers within a general hospital and include physician specialists; others are freestanding specialty clinics and outpatient facility joint ventures between hospitals and physicians. An increasing number of physician-owned ambulatory specialty facilities also aims to attract consumers who seek more choice of care. Specialty service-line organization in the outpatient sector reflects the long-standing specialization of physicians. Now joining ambulatory surgery centers are a myriad of facilities dedicated to diagnostic imaging, sleep disorders, cosmetic surgery, radiotherapy, cancer chemotherapy, peripheral vascular disease, gastrointestinal endoscopy, coronary care units, and so on. The extent to which service-line development actually reorganizes care varies; it could comprise completely separate profit centers and freestanding units that support the rest of a hospital, or it could comprise purely marketing exercises that rebrand and administer special service lines within general hospitals.[26]

These niche centers and their associated physicians have escalated competition over control of specialty services, siphoning off the most lucrative patients and procedures. Less profitable services

25. Devers, Brewster, and Casalino, "Changes in Hospital Competitive Strategy," 460.

26. Berenson, Bodenheimer, and Pham, "Specialty-Service Lines," w339.

are then relegated to general medical hospitals, who subsequently experience decreased revenues even as they must find ways to subsidize the provision of uncompensated care.[27] Single-specialty clinics that focus on fewer profitable services may be able to "provide many amenities and take market share away from community hospitals struggling to provide and cross-subsidize a wide range of general services."[28] Supporters of specialty hospitals and clinics assert that increased choices available to health care purchasers will result in a rise in the total amount of health care available to the population; inequalities exacerbated by these facilities are permissible under the proviso of increasing competition to improve quality of care and lower costs.[29] However, health care markets serve those who can afford to purchase services and erode the cross-subsidies that have financed access to care in the United States. Large elite nonprofit general hospitals have responded to service-line competition by recouping revenue losses from out-migrated services and uncompensated care by raising prices and volumes of specialty-line services as well as locking in specialist physician admissions to induce demand for services.[30] Academic medical centers—forced to compete with often more efficient private hospitals and specialty clinics—have assiduously courted patients from overseas in order to improve their financial edge because the care of overseas patients is not subject to Medicare and Medicaid restrictions or insurance reimbursement requirements. "Super hospitals" seek to extend their international clientele and form alliances with civic-oriented and business organizations to support the needs of patients travel-

27. Nelson and Wolf-Powers, "Chains and Ladders," 34.

28. Devers, Brewster, and Casalino, "Changes in Hospital Competitive Strategy," 464.

29. Robert A. Berenson, Gloria J. Bazzoli, and Melanie Au, "Do Specialty Hospitals Promote Price Competition?," Issue Brief 103, *Center for Studying Health System Change,* January 2006, http://www.hschange.org/CONTENT/816/.

30. Berenson, Bodenheimer, and Pham, "Specialty-Service Lines," w342; Nelson, "Are Hospitals an Export Industry?," 251.

ing overseas and to create different "catchment areas" that target specific populations, in some cases reaching global dimensions.[31]

American hospitals offer a unique blend of medical research and innovative clinical techniques. Building on international awareness of U.S. medical expertise, an array of hospitals now market luxury primary care clinics to recruit wealthy foreign patients, including Massachusetts General Hospital, New York Presbyterian, the University of Miami, and the University of California, San Francisco. Hospitals branch out to offer hospitality services and joint ventures, enlisting spectacular architecture and exclusive amenities. Given that the overall structure of the U.S. health care system favors corporations and high-technology products and services, the pursuit of global architectural boosterism and technologic innovation by these medical institutions requires dramatic capital expenditures that help drive up the overall cost of health care worldwide.[32] The strategy also promotes an ideology of demand-driven consumer health satisfaction and the opportunity to opt for the best, most exclusive care tied to the latest medical technologies and services as a way to ensure quality. Executive health programs at leading hospitals, for example, organize corporate packages of health physicals that function like visits to a spa. Nearly three thousand individuals visit the Mayo Clinic each year for a two- or three-day itinerary of customized and comprehensive services at multiple global locations. In addition to cardiovascular counseling, lifestyle assessment, and in-depth, one-on-one review by a personal executive health physician, patients have access to amenities ranging from business lounges to Botox.

To reach international patients, hospitals have developed international hospitality organizations that secure referrals and generate

31. Andrea A. Cortinois, Sarah Downey, Tom Closson, and Alejandro R. Jadad, "Hospitals in a Globalized World: A View From Canada," *HealthcarePapers* 4, no. 2 (2003): 23.

32. Waitzkin, *Medicine and Public Health,* 40.

revenue to subsidize hospital teaching and research programs.[33] The Cleveland Clinic's main campus, for instance, showcases a posh international center with interpreter services and foreign newspapers, special diets, convenient transportation, insurance assistance, and infrastructure dedicated to obtaining preadmission overseas records. The clinic also owns several hotels managed by the Cleveland Clinic InterContinental Hotel Group, which advertises internationally and attracts patients via airline magazines, hospital exchange programs, embassy contacts, corporate agreements, and listings in international medical directories. Hospitals sign cooperative agreements to collaborate on patient referrals, physician visits, medical education, and administrative training. They also initiate separate start-up companies or special international service centers that adapt procedures and workflows to assist international clients. The International Program at Johns Hopkins Hospital successfully ballooned the international patient population from five hundred before 1994 to more than seven thousand by 1998, and Johns Hopkins Medicine International—a for-profit venture jointly owned by JHU and Johns Hopkins Medicine—forms strategic overseas partnerships that facilitate medical tourism.[34] Additionally, hospital links to embassies and medical travel intermediaries—for example, Companion Global Healthcare and International Patient Services—curate a prequalified selection of hospitals and advise on care options, set up appointments in U.S. hospitals, and essentially operate as specialized travel agents.[35]

A focus on user experience and architectural spectacle tied to wellness pervades these efforts to attract international clientele

33. Olivia F. Lee and Tim R. V. Davis, "International Patients: A Lucrative Market for U.S. Hospitals," *Health Marketing Quarterly* 22, no. 1 (2004): 51.

34. John J. Hutchins, "Bringing International Patients to American Hospitals: The Johns Hopkins Perspective," *Managed Care Quarterly* 6, no. 3 (1998): 22, 24.

35. Herrick, "Medical Tourism," 6; Lee and Davis, "International Patients," 50.

and patients able to afford specialty services. As the top-ranked and largest private medical center in the United States, the Mayo Medical Center's main campus in Rochester, Minnesota, features the acclaimed Leslie and Susan Gonda Building, designed by Ellerbe Becket and Cesar Pelli & Associates. Constructed in 2000–2001, the Gonda building's northern section incorporates a flowing curtain wall system with granite spandrel and column panels. A seven-story skyway connects the north side of the building to another Mayo building across the street, while a stone-clad elevator lifts people up the building's twenty-one floors—soon to be expanded by an additional eleven floors.[36] With a marble-sheathed lobby overlooking a sunken garden, the building is also fused to another Ellerbe creation, the Mayo Building (1954), trimmed with rose-tinted windows and a marble exterior.[37] The Mayo campus and Rochester's outer districts contain numerous other architectural trophies from Franklin Ellerbe, Frank Lloyd Wright, and Eero Saarinen, revealing long-standing efforts to foster monumental therapeutic design attractions.[38]

Specialty clinics like the Cleveland Clinic Lou Ruvo Center for Brain Health in Las Vegas, Nevada, enlist architectural boosterism to challenge the clinical atmosphere altogether, supporting specialized research and care through spectacular fundraising events. Opened in 2010 in the sixty-one-acre Symphony Park, the outpatient treatment center for Alzheimer disease, Parkinson disease, Huntington disease, multiple sclerosis, and ALS was designed by architect Frank Gehry and comprises two buildings joined by a

---

36. Vertical Access, "Project Profile: Gonda Building, Mayo Clinic Rochester, MN," accessed November 7, 2022, https://vertical-access.com/wp-content/uploads/2016/06/gonda_building_mayo_clinic.pdf; Christopher Snowbeck, "Mayo Expansion Would Create Rochester's Tallest Building," *StarTribune,* September 18, 2018, https://www.startribune.com/mayo-plans-190m-building-expansion-in-rochester/493592401/.

37. Joel Hoekstra, "Rochester: A Design Tour," accessed November 7, 2022, https://www.aia-mn.org/rochester-design-tour/.

38. Hoekstra, "Rochester."

steel trellis shading an outdoor patio. Costing $80–100 million, the approximately 65,000-square-foot complex is draped with mountainous metal-clad skin, faced with shingled panels, and punctured by a grid of different-size windows.[39] The metal wrapper forms a freestanding structure that envelops a soaring sculptural volume with a cathedral-like event space: the Life Activity Center. Patients follow a breezeway to the entrance of the separate four-story medical building of jumbled boxy forms in white stucco and glass that houses exam rooms, offices, research center, and the nonprofit Keep Memory Alive headquarters.[40] Boasting 65,000 hours of engineering, with 199 windows (none alike) and 18,000 stainless steel shingles (each cut to unique measurements), the building projects an image of its own exorbitant cost in a bid to draw patients and raise further funds.[41]

Joint ventures and global medical hubs extend elite U.S. hospital operations and clinical practices into global trade circuits, with locations and architecture that network medical expertise and prestige for elite medical tourism and trade. Over three dozen U.S. hospitals and health systems now operate overseas. Alliances vary from medical school exchanges to transnational jointly managed clinics. For example, Harvard Medical International works with Wockhardt Hospitals Group in India; the Children's Hospital of Philadelphia coordinates with the United Arab Emirates (UAE) and Massachusetts

39. Ridhika Naidoo, "Frank Gehry: The Cleveland Clinic Lou Ruvo Center for Brain Health," *Design Boom,* May 28, 2010, https://www.designboom.com/architecture/frank-gehry-the-cleveland-clinic-lou-ruvo-center-for-brain-health/; Joseph Giovannini, "Cleveland Clinic Lou Ruvo Center for Brain Health," *Architect Magazine,* April 7, 2011, https://www.architectmagazine.com/design/buildings/cleveland-clinic-lou-ruvo-center-for-brain-health_o.

40. David Basulto, "Cleveland Clinic Lou Ruvo Center for Brain Health/Frank Gehry," *ArchDaily*, June 22, 2010, https://www.archdaily.com/65609/center-for-brain-health.

41. Keep Memory Alive, "Tour Our Frank Gehry Designed Campus," accessed November 7, 2022, https://www.keepmemoryalive.org/our-campus/tour-our-frank-gehry-designed-campus.

General Hospital with Jiahui Health, a private system in Shanghai; and Miami Beach's Mount Sinai Medical Center has partnered with hospitals in Guatemala and the Dominican Republic.[42] Beyond consulting with foreign companies, these partnerships can involve directly investing in a foreign hospital facility via full or partial ownership, or establishing a management contract for all or some hospital functions without ownership interest.[43] In some cases, prestigious American universities or health care systems open branches where they are directly responsible for providing care and linking activities of medical research, education, business, and clinical treatment in a centralized medical hub. A missionary ideology of advancing research and education internationally, as well as improving clinical services and quality, pervades these competing medical spheres of influence. The developmentalist drive to set new global standards and "give back to the world" articulates with efforts to elevate one's brand and international profile, commercialize intellectual property, and network lab services, analytics, protocols, and virtual products. The transnational operations of U.S. hospital systems extend Western biomedical concepts of health and competition while seeking international talent, treatments, research, technologies, and pharmaceuticals in order to boost revenue.[44] Even as they index the historical vestiges of Western colonial legacies, these medical entrepôts reconfigure center–periphery relations by performing globality in branded networks within the political economy of empire and international public health.[45]

42. Lee and Davis, "International Patients," 47.

43. Jacqueline S. Zinn, Roger J. Kashlak, and Edward R. Balotsky, "Selecting International Markets: Lessons from For-Profit Hospitals," *Hospital and Health Services Administration* 39, no. 1 (1994): 23.

44. Altaf Virani, Adam M. Wellstead, and Michael Howlett, "The North–South Policy Divide in Transnational Healthcare: A Comparative Review of Policy Research on Medical Tourism," *Globalization and Health* 16, no. 37 (2020): 12.

45. Eng-Beng Lim, "Performing the Global University," *Social Text* 27, no. 4 (2009): 28–29.

The over $14 billion University of Pittsburgh Medical Center (UPMC) exemplifies the international orientation and competitive market for specialty clinic outposts. UPMC International has aggressively established multiple cancer treatment centers in the United States, Ireland, and Italy.[46] In Italy, UPMC formed a joint public–private partnership with the region of Sicily and local hospitals to establish a leading European transplantation center, where they perform thousands of transplantations, clinical therapies, and treatment alternatives since its establishment in 1997.[47] The Palermo-based partnership further established the Cell Factory—laboratories that produce cells to treat end-stage organ failure.[48] UPMC also bought a stake in the Chianciano Spa in Tuscany to offer personalized diagnostic screenings and procedures, a medical wellness center, and healthy lifestyle programs in connection to the spa's thermal water therapies.[49] In Ireland, UPMC took over the operations of the largest private hospital in the southeast of the country and expanded UPMC Sports Medicine to its first overseas clinic location in Waterford to treat athletes and active people. In 2019, UPMC Kildare Hospital entered a partnership with the largest ophthalmology service in Ireland—the Institute of Eye Surgery—to create a national Ophthalmology Network of Excellence that features the cutting-edge research and clinical trials of world-renowned UPMC-based Dr. José-Alain Sahel to prevent and cure blindness.[50] That same year, UPMC signed an agreement with the

46. Refer to the UPMC International website, accessed November 7, 2022, https://www.upmc.com/about/international-services.

47. UPMC, "Instituto Mediterraneo per i Trapianti e Terapie ad Alta Specializzazione (ISMETT)," accessed November 7, 2022, https://www.upmc.com/about/international-services/locations/italy.

48. Istituto di Ricovero e Cura a Carattere Scientifico, "Regenerative Medicine and Cellular Therapies Unit," November 7, 2022, https://www.ismett.edu/en/regenerative-medicine-and-cellular-therapies-unit/.

49. UPMC Institute for Health Chianciano Terme, accessed November 7, 2022, https://www.upmcchianciano.it/.

50. UPMC International, "Locations and Partnerships: Ireland," accessed November 7, 2022, https://www.upmc.com/about/international-services/locations/ireland.

China-based multinational conglomerate Wanda Group—one of the world's largest real estate, film, children's entertainment, sports, and tourism companies—to jointly build and operate multiple hospitals in China, with UPMC providing expertise in hospital design, procedures, and management best practices.[51] In a strategic entrance into Eurasia, UPMC also works with Nazarbayev University to establish Kazakhstan's first fully integrated academic medical center, upgrading the teaching hospital and anticipating greater profit margins than U.S. hospitals.[52]

The academic medical teaching and research arm of JHU, the Johns Hopkins School of Medicine, has joined hands with big oil by inaugurating a joint project with the energy and integrated global petrochemicals company Saudi Aramco. Collaborating in 2013 to create the first-of-its-kind health care joint venture, Johns Hopkins Aramco Healthcare serves Aramco employees and their descendants and retirees, who all receive care free of charge. In addition to owning equity in the joint venture, Johns Hopkins provides education, training, and clinical programming; operations management and support; and direct clinical care by rotating Johns Hopkins faculty in subspecialties. Patients are seen at Dhahran Health Center, a 330-bed tertiary care hospital, as well as other satellite outpatient facilities.[53] The Dhahran primary care clinic specializes in cardiac surgery, cardiac rehabilitation, com-

51. UPMC International, "Locations and Partnerships: China," accessed November 7, 2022, https://www.upmc.com/about/international-services/locations/china.

52. UPMC International, "Locations and Partnerships: Kazakhstan," accessed November 7, 2022, https://www.upmc.com/about/international-al-services/locations/kazakhstan.

53. Johns Hopkins Medicine International, "Johns Hopkins Aramco Healthcare," accessed November 7, 2022, https://www.hopkinsmedicine.org/international/health-care-consulting/our-clients/emea/johns_hopkins_aramco_healthcare.html; Johns Hopkins Aramco Healthcare, "Johns Hopkins Aramco Healthcare—Our History," accessed November 7, 2022, https://www.jhah.com/en/about-us.

plex electrophysiology, palliative care, endovascular therapies, and noninvasive imaging; it also offers weight management and smoking cessation programs.[54] The facility features an automated pharmacy, a children's play area, a sanctuary garden, and the new patient-centered Suite Six, which places the patient at the center of care: medical services largely take place in one room with a care team, a desirable alternative to making patients navigate the complex institution.[55] The website and promotional materials, which are central to marketing Johns Hopkins Aramco Healthcare, plot a timeline of innovative medical practices that parallel drilling operations in Saudi Arabia, starting with a single doctor in 1936 and establishing the need for a hospital and pharmacy to address employees' medical needs attendant to refinery establishment. The narrative progresses with Aramco's accreditation success and placement of Saudi students in top U.S. medical schools, including Harvard, Tulane, and the University of Alabama, and peaks with the 2013 partnership that boasts the only health system outside of the United States that officially bears the Johns Hopkins name.[56]

Similarly, the largest health care network in the UAE, Abu Dhabi Health Services Company (SEHA), has partnered with the Mayo Clinic on the joint operation of one of the UAE's largest hospitals for patients with complex medical conditions, now known as Mayo Clinic Sheikh Shakhbout Medical City.[57] With collaborative ventures on seven continents, the Mayo Clinic entered the Middle East as a shareholder in the new operating company, thus marking a new type of international health care relationship in the UAE with the company/SEHA that owns and operates all of the public hospitals and

54. Johns Hopkins Aramco Healthcare, "Specialty Care," accessed November 7, 2022, https://www.jhah.com/en/care-services/specialty-care.

55. Johns Hopkins Aramco Healthcare, *Well*Being, April 2017, https://www.jhah.com/media/2248/english-wellbeing-april-2017.pdf, 4.

56. Johns Hopkins Aramco Healthcare, "Johns Hopkins Aramco Healthcare—Our History."

57. The facility replaces the existing Al Mafraq Hospital.

clinics in the emirate of Abu Dhabi.[58] After the 2019 development agreement, the 3.2 million square foot, multispecialty, state-of-the-art hospital will be staffed with more than four hundred internationally trained physicians and will invest in medical technology to promote advanced diagnostics, specialized procedures for arteries and burns, and less invasive techniques, all complemented by a new medical research center designed to promote comprehensive interdisciplinary learning.[59] The $817 million facility features four towers with patient rooms, each of which offers views of the campus and access to rooftop gardens; in addition, designated floors offer enhanced privacy, with two presidential suites and thirty-six VIP suites.[60] Mayo Clinic International roots the project in the legacy of its founders—Will and Charlie Mayo—who traveled the globe and established Mayo's legacy as an international organization that "learns from others and shares knowledge and expertise to benefit patients."[61] Mayo Clinic faculty will now supervise the clinical training of Gulf Medical University students at the medical complex in order to strengthen medical education, professional development, and clinical research.[62]

The Cleveland Clinic has taken further steps to open its own independent medical hubs in other countries, prominently using

58. Karl Oestreich, "SEHA, Mayo Clinic Enter Joint Venture to Operate Sheikh Shakhbout Medical City," *Mayo Clinic News Network,* November 24, 2019, https://newsnetwork.mayoclinic.org/discussion/seha-mayo-clinic-enter-joint-venture-to-operate-sheikh-shakhbout-medical-city/.

59. Oestreich, "SEHA, Mayo Clinic Enter Joint Venture."

60. Anne DiNardo, "Sheikh Shakhbout Medical City," *Healthcare Design Magazine,* March 24, 2020, https://healthcaredesignmagazine.com/projects/acute-care/photo-tour-sheikh-shakhbout-medical-city/.

61. G. Anton Decker, MBBCh, president of Mayo Clinic International, quoted in Oestreich, "SEHA, Mayo Clinic Enter Joint Venture."

62. Gulf Medical University, "Gulf Medical University Tie Up with Sheikh Shakhbout Medical City, Mayo Clinic, Abu Dhabi," accessed November 7, 2022, https://gmu.ac.ae/gulf-medical-university-tie-up-with-sheikh-shakhbout-medical-city-mayo-clinic-abu-dhabi-in-clinical-training-and-cancer-research/.

its name on buildings, signs, and lab coats. Joining Cleveland Clinic Canada in downtown Toronto (2006), Cleveland Clinic London began welcoming patients in March 2022. Located across the street from Buckingham Palace, the clinic operates without a local partner and offers elective surgeries for the privately insured. Emergency services are not planned, as they are not required, nor considered to be financially lucrative. Before the venture, in 2015, the Cleveland Clinic developed the multispecialty Cleveland Clinic Abu Dhabi in the heart of the UAE city's new central business district on Al Maryah Island. Collaboratively planned with the government-owned Mubadala Development company, the twenty-three-acre facility extends the U.S.-based Cleveland Clinic's model of care to 364 beds (expandable to 490 beds), five clinical floors, three diagnostic and treatment levels, and thirteen floors of critical and acute care inpatient units.[63] The clinic and each of its specialized care areas were designed with the input of more than three hundred physicians and clinical personnel, as well as hundreds of architects, planners, and interior designers.[64] The clinic, which cost approximately $2.5 billion, holds the title of the largest structural steel building in the UAE and has received accolades for blurring the line between hospital and luxury hotel. The facility displays distinctive diamond glazing and a glowing double-skinned patient tower; sleek glass walkways connect inpatient spaces with a 340-exam-room outpatient clinic, 210 faculty offices, conference center, simulation center, and administration building. Clad in perforated and corrugated metal skin, the highly textured surface of the complex's podium refracts sunlight and is capped by a flowing glass structure that illuminates the metal base at night with LEDs that create a moiré

63. Elizabeth Evitts Dickinson, "Global Hospitals: The Cleveland Clinic Abu Dhabi," *Architect Magazine,* February 16, 2010, https://www. architectmagazine.com/design/buildings/global-hospitals-the-cleveland-clinic-abu-dhabi_o.

64. "Cleveland Clinic Brings World-Class Care to Abu Dhabi," *HDR Inc.,* accessed November 7, 2022, https://www.hdrinc.com/portfolio/cleveland-clinic-abu-dhabi.

effect.[65] Patients enter a lobby wrapped in marble, stone, and wood, with modern interiors, verdant gardens, and expansive common spaces, including an upscale retail gallery overlooking the city. The color palette riffs on the surrounding natural elements: glass echoes the radiant turquoise of the gulf's waters, while onyx and an array of neutral tones reference the arid landscape. Interior patterns and motifs invest in a burgeoning vernacular of arabesque patterned screen elements; indoor water features provide white noise to calm patients.[66] Patient rooms are intentionally designed with large family spaces and abundant windows with views of lush rooftop gardens and the Arabian Sea. The exclusive hospital features private suites for VIPs and a floor reserved for the royal family, with a secure entry, private elevator access, and private quarters for the patient's doctors. Its opening drew more than five thousand physicians from around the world to apply for the initial 175 doctor positions in the hospital, with 80 percent of the successful applicants trained in the United States and the rest in Europe.[67]

While such transnational branches and joint ventures may facilitate international education, cross-cultural understanding, and a global medical commons, they also extract considerable resources, and their role as a domestic welfare and development strategy is debatable. International revenues can improve health care standards and reinvest in local economies and cities. However, these profits remain a small portion of institutional portfolios and do not curb costs.[68] Furthermore, this burgeoning network of medical entrepôts

65. Sebastian Jordana, "Cleveland Clinic Abu Dhabi/HDR," *Archdaily. com,* November 12, 2012, https://www.archdaily.com/292167/in-progress-cleveland-clinic-abu-dhabi-hdr-architecture.

66. Jordana, "Cleveland Clinic Abu Dhabi/HDR."

67. Jennifer Bell, "Inside Cleveland Clinic Abu Dhabi: 5,500 Doctors Apply for 175 Positions," *National News UAE,* June 28, 2014, https://www. thenationalnews.com/uae/health/inside-cleveland-clinic-abu-dhabi-5-500-doctors-apply-for-175-positions-1.308836.

68. Jordan Rau, "Hemmed in at Home, Nonprofit Hospitals Look for Profits Abroad," *KHN.org,* June 22, 2021, https://khn.org/news/article/hemmed-in-at-home-nonprofit-hospitals-look-for-profits-abroad/.

of American health care depends on domestic extraction, burdening public resources and thriving on land grabs and real estate developments. Rather than addressing structural issues that limit health care access and coverage, U.S. policy has focused more on creating transnational brand extension and management arrangements, global networks of accredited health care providers, and cross-border insurance mechanisms to support overseas treatment.[69] U.S. for-profit entities and nonprofits that function like for-profits—hospital systems, health maintenance organizations, and pharmaceutical and biotechnology companies—extend internationally to find new revenue streams, address labor shortages, and cut costs. They increasingly outsource business functions, found technology transfer offices, establish start-ups and incubators, and become entrepreneurial exporters of management consulting, real estate, and other practices perceived to fuel innovation. The increasing amount of for-profit care options creates a predatory business climate: for-profit success depends on betting against public systems in other countries and banking on private alternatives to taxpayer-funded health systems.

This incursion of market-driven foreign private health services challenges the territorial governance of health care. Governments partly derive their political legitimacy from ensuring the welfare of their national populations; indeed, "entitlement to receive health care and responsibility to financially contribute to the health system that provides such care, therefore, are frequently considered part of a broader package of national membership."[70] However, the penetration of private enterprises into national health sectors eliminates the prioritization of domestic providers. In the United States, the strategy of using international for-profit operations to subsidize local development and research/teaching missions per-

69. Virani, Wellstead, and Howlett, "North–South Policy Divide," 11.
70. Meghann Ormond and Neil Lunt, "Transnational Medical Travel: Patient Mobility, Shifting Health System Entitlements and Attachments," *Journal of Ethnic and Migration Studies* 46, no. 20 (2020): 4179.

versely poaches patients from national health care systems overseas while doing nothing for the approximately 27.5 million of the population without health insurance.[71] The globalization of American health care has privileged profit over health coverage. Where U.S. hospitals open overseas hubs, they support international patient prospecting and global circuits of trade in hospitality services that inflate costs, compound climate change, and further divide elites from the poor. There is nothing inherently wrong with many of the special health services examined here; wellness and nutrition programs, for example, focus on everyday health and environmental awareness. However, the political-economic positioning of such services reveals the massive discrepancies of health attendant to this transnational U.S. medical development complex. Elite hospital systems offer specialty private care through increasingly ambiguous governance; they engage in predatory relations with overseas national health care systems while outperforming large U.S. urban hospitals, which are left to subsidize uncompensated care through specialty services that can no longer compete financially. Telemedicine adds further levels of complexity to governing such transnational practices—especially their environmental impact and relationship to place-based labor.

The detrimental consequences of neoliberal global trade agreements and the resource-intensive domestic operations of U.S. hospitals should raise alarm over the environmental governance of this burgeoning transnational medical development complex. In response to the damaging environmental effects, myriad organizations have emerged to "green" U.S. health care and advocate regulatory and social responsibility–based actions. These efforts have targeted hospitals for emissions reductions as a means to decrease the 6.7 to 7 million annual fatalities and countless other health problems estimated to result from poor ambient air quality worldwide. Reducing

71. U.S. Census Bureau, "Health Insurance Coverage in the United States: 2018," November 8, 2019, https://www.census.gov/library/publications/2019/demo/p60-267.html.

emissions also seeks to lower the mounting 34,000 annual cancer cases in the United States attributable to occupational and environmental exposures.[72] Other initiatives seek healthy, locally sourced food in hospital cafeterias and food service; sustainable local furniture, bedding, and supplies; and safer alternatives for pest management, cleaning, disinfection, mercury elimination, and hazardous waste removal. While there are clear benefits to this sustainability drive, we also see the treatment of the environment as a mere staging ground for operational cost-effectiveness and design efficiencies, rather than addressing the globalizing health care system's active role in perpetuating environmental inequality, thus reinforcing the specialized vertical structure of ineffective health systems while failing to improve access to care. Sustainability in health care is not equated with public socialized health but instead with technical enhancements to the highly inequitable profit-oriented acute care and privatized insurance, or with reducing "government waste" by lowering public funding and implementing further medical "deservingness" qualifications in Medicare and especially Medicaid.

Environmental greening initiatives at the global scale mirror the language used in U.S. brownfield land conversions. Both impose a certain model of health justified in terms of improvement—bettering a contaminated land parcel or resource-intensive building, or tapping into an untouched market. Yet as previously discussed, hospital systems themselves contribute to blight and intentionally expand into environmentally vulnerable places; they exacerbate the environmental health hazards and risks experienced by populations in

72. Figures were derived from the Institute for Health Metrics Evaluation "Global Burden of Disease Study" of 2019 (latest data collected in 2021) and World Health Organization analysis of 2016 (latest data collected in 2021), as cited by Max Roser, "Data Review: How Many People Die from Air Pollution?," *Our World in Data,* November 25, 2021, https://ourworldindata.org/data-review-air-pollution-deaths. The estimated number of deaths from cancer attributable to occupational and environmental exposures has been controversial. The figure quoted is from Eckelman and Sherman, "Environmental Impacts," 10.

these places, especially via their interactions with labor and service lines that support elites. The transnational hospitality and service extensions of U.S. hospitals and medical centers financially depend on the colonial operations of these domestic medical brownfields to underwrite their overseas branches and enlist sustainability indicators to buttress their competitive growth. Thus, however ostensibly "good" these sustainability measures appear, they also greenwash systemic issues of structural inequality, violence, land dispossession, and public sector predation.

Cleveland Clinic Abu Dhabi emblematizes the contradictory implementation of sustainability in the context of proliferating specialty clinics, executive health programs, and joint ventures that extend patient catchment areas and stoke a globalizing medical arms race. The clinic seeks to green its development aesthetics to the extent that international accounting for adverse impacts on climate has become a new "zero-waste" frontier. Even as the high-end hospital demands intense resources—which run the gamut from masses of concrete and steel in its construction to energy-intensive HVAC systems and medical waste streams—the facility was awarded a Gold sustainability certificate for new construction by the most widely used green building rating system: Leadership in Energy and Environmental Design, better known as LEED. It became one of the first hospitals in the Middle East and North Africa region to use a greenhouse gas tool to log all of its greenhouse gas emissions. It has implemented countless waste elimination measures, including reducing reliance on desalination plants, using solar water heaters, and converting food waste into compost for the hospital's gardens.[73] Yet it has focused exclusively on building efficiencies in a closed ecology; it has created a profitable loop of the hospital's waste and wastefulness, ignoring the complex material geographies

73. "Cleveland Clinic Abu Dhabi Pushes to be 'Greenest' Hospital in GCC," press release, *Zawya.com,* April 24, 2019, https://www.zawya.com/mena/en/press-releases/story/Cleveland_Clinic_Abu_Dhabi_pushes_to_be_Greenest_Hospital_in_GCC-ZAWYA20190424072012/.

upstream and downstream of the facility and the inequities fueled by its billion-dollar existence. The political economic positioning of the Cleveland Clinic system and its extensions into global circuits of capital and medical tourism, combined with the adverse environmental racism of its domestic operations, contribute to vastly inequitable territorial stratification of health and disease burden. The absurdity of its greening initiatives in the context of austerity, home foreclosures, and Covid devastation at its U.S. home base of Cleveland further underscores how ameliorating the emissions of medical hospitality services and clinical practices at the Abu Dhabi campus decenters care and politics by dividing biomedical and technological practices from socioecological issues.

Under the sign of sustainability, "green" functions as a settler-colonial ideology that allows for the technocratic disavowal of the health care system's harmful impacts. While claiming benefits trickle down, medical joint ventures and global hubs extend the domestically extractive processes of U.S. hospitals transnationally, further dividing the medical haves from the have-nots, thus advancing health colonialism. The colonial relations of development that underpin U.S. medical outposts globalize profit-oriented private acute care and perpetuate tautologies of racial violence along a global color line.[74] The moralizing discourse of medical progress and educational mission—coupled with architectural spectacles of sustainability—severs the fundamental tenet of health care practice, do no harm, from considerations of the active role of the U.S. health care system in socioenvironmental and political-economic violence. As such, it is imperative to weigh the harm of policies that rely on determinations of blight and their anchoring of transnational speculative development projects that further intensify health, environmental, and geopolitical inequalities.

74. W. E. B. Du Bois, "Prospect of a World without Racial Conflict," *American Journal of Sociology* 49, no. 5 (1944): 452.

Conclusion: Decolonizing Health

THE COVID-19 PANDEMIC exposed vulnerabilities and failures endemic to U.S. health care. It dramatically revealed the system's unsustainability when revenue-generating elective procedures were halted to meet the demand for ICU beds and other necessary equipment, leading to hospital and clinic closures when they were needed most.[1] The promise of future returns and trickle-down benefits collapsed as the immediate emergency suspended the costly elective procedures that subsidize welfare. The United States has the lowest return on life expectancy for health care expenditure, with individuals receiving low-quality care compared to other high-income countries.[2] Many Americans cannot afford private health coverage or cannot meet the eligibility requirements of public health programs, so they cannot access quality health care, health insurance, or positive health outcomes. Nor is quality care guaran-

1. Nick Culbertson, "How Hospitals are Handling Compliance in a Resource-Constrained Environment," *Forbes,* December 7, 2020, https://www.forbes.com/sites/forbestechcouncil/2020/12/07/how-hospitals-are-handling-compliance-in-a-resource-constrained-environment/?sh=11160e672c77.

2. Roosa Tikkanen and Melinda K. Abrams, "U.S. Health Care from a Global Perspective, 2019: Higher Spending, Worse Outcomes?," Issue Brief, *Commonwealth Fund,* January 30, 2020, https://www.commonwealthfund.org/publications/issue-briefs/2020/jan/us-health-care-global-perspective-2019.

teed or evenly distributed for the insured. Such fissures in health and access to health care existed long before the pandemic and have been devastatingly intensified by it, as seen in the relentless numbers of deaths reflected on Covid dashboards.

Chapter 3 touched on technocratic efforts to "green" health care that decenter the politics of care and further divide biomedical and socioecological issues under the sign of sustainability. Technological fixes and spectacles of sustainability can eclipse the role of American health care in perpetuating power relations of debt, dependency, and medical inequality that sustain global health apartheid. This is especially true with respect to the extraction of health care labor. The term "green" is equated with renewable energy production, environmental management and conservation, and operational efficiencies that save on resources; it does not necessarily designate jobs that support and preserve health, well-being, culture, intergenerational equity, and the land and ecologies on which we rely.[3] Health care sector green projects—including the laudable and necessary goal of reducing energy consumption and emissions—will perpetuate colonial relations with land and labor across a global color line if social transformation is not tied to energy transition. Decarbonization efforts should strive to decolonize biomedicine— and its underwriting of the property system, debt, and devaluation of care work—in favor of more equitable and collective provisioning for everyday good lives and good deaths.

Numerous initiatives at international aid organizations, universities, and schools of public health have advocated for decolonizing global health and addressing power inequities.[4] This movement

3. Lenore Palladino and Rhianna Gunn-Wright, "Care and Climate: Understanding the Policy Intersections—A Feminist Green New Deal Coalition Brief," *Feminist Green New Deal*, April 2021, http://feministgreen-newdeal.com/wp-content/uploads/2021/04/FemGND-IssueBrief-Draft7-Apr15.pdf, 15.

4. Zeinabou Niamé Daffé, Yodeline Guillaume, and Louise C. Ivers, "Anti-racism and Anti-colonialism Praxis in Global Health—Reflection and Action for Practitioners in U.S. Academic Medical Centers," *American Journal of Tropical Medicine and Hygiene* 105, no. 3 (2021): 557.

is not new, of course; the intellectual, political, and other labor of communities engaged in high-intensity struggle have developed these critiques as a matter of survival.[5] Efforts to acknowledge and respond to these struggles within health fields have made it common practice to refer to what is termed "social determinants of health," to mark the inequitable conditions of health. However, as Ruha Benjamin, Kim Gallon, and other Black feminist scholars and data ethicists have argued, reliance on quantitative approaches to substantiate the social contexts of health can lead to the datafication of disease, illness, injury, and death—and not necessarily any social change. Exemplifying this, pandemic representations of health demographics have had the effect of reifying nonwhite race as marked for death.[6] Racist tautologies wedded to a technocratic worldview are a form of ongoing coloniality. Although colonialism is frequently named as a social determinant of health, colonization is not merely a variable or an isolated historical event. Rather, it is one of developing and unremitting unequal relationships with negative effects on health.[7] Colonial processes continue to shape medicine and health care—their material and epistemological foundations, organization, and practices.

This book has pursued an analytic shift from colonialism as a social determinant of health to the active role of U.S. health care in colonialism. The critique is not intended to rebuke the sacrifices and

5. Sharon Stein, "What Can Decolonial and Abolitionist Critiques Teach the Field of Higher Education?," *Review of Higher Education* 44, no. 3 (2021): 391.

6. Ruha Benjamin, "Black Skin, White Masks: Racism, Vulnerability and Refuting Black Pathology," video, 30:48, Department of African American Studies, Princeton University, April 15, 2020, https://aas.princeton.edu/news/black-skin-white-masks-racism-vulnerability-refuting-black-pathology; Kim Gallon, "A Review of Covid-19 Intersectional Data Decision-making: A Call for Black Feminist Data Analytics, Part I," *Covid Black*, September 18, 2020, https://covidblack.medium.com/a-review-of-covid-19-intersectional-data-decision-making-a-call-for-black-feminist-data-analytics-da8e12bc4a6b.

7. Czyzewski, "Colonialism," 10.

intentions of health care workers across the professional spectrum. It apprehends the contributions and constitutive function of the U.S. health care industry and medical institutions in ongoing health colonialism—that is, sociospatial domination and exploitation, along with the ideological frameworks, logics, and mythologies that underpin this, to produce unequal life conditions, diminished livelihoods, and premature death. Health colonialism takes many forms: devaluation and repression of care work; infiltration of substandard for-profit care in BIPOC communities; and chronic underfunding, fragmentation, and privatization of local health care systems and public hospitals. I have examined health colonialism in terms of the structural violence of U.S. health care, specifically its property frontiers and pedagogies of urban redevelopment and educational mission. The analysis considers the ways that biomedicine colonizes space with health impacts, focusing on the land practices of several prestigious nonprofit hospitals and medical centers within a system that prioritizes profitability and specialized acute care over everyday collective forms of health. To denaturalize the land relations of these institutions, I foreground waste colonialism and the way articulations of waste and race entrench settler and anti-Black domination in order to underscore the noninnocent geographical foundations of U.S. biomedicine. I use the case of racial-capitalist brownfields to open up a broader view of land confiscation within the context of the U.S. settler-colonial property frontier: not only is pollution used as a technique to dispossess, but also the adaptable colonial logic of wasteland extends to the land pedagogies of blight and public use to position inhabitants as lacking "the liberal capitalist insights and technological know-how to properly occupy a city."[8] U.S. health care institutions perpetrate white liberal property violence via the colonial occupation and pollution of land that displace communities and strip assets from domestic development zones.

8. Paperson, "Ghetto Land Pedagogy," 120.

When we place brick-and-mortar hospitals within the everyday political economy of real estate development practices, we see extensive divisions among these key health care institutions and the way that some engage in spatial and fiscal eminent domain through land dispossession, clearance, and gentrification. U.S. urban policies have driven hospitals toward property-oriented growth as part of racially oppressive public-policy responses to urban unrest. In turn, U.S. health policies have supported a model of private health care strongholds with emergency services and police forces in the context of general medical scarcity for poor and uninsured people. The property-based orientation of these imbricated policies mobilizes an elastic frontier of urban blight and colonial land grabs in the name of revitalization, sustainability, community development, and education. Pro-growth, pro-development urban anchor policies have secured massive biomedical complexes that actively create blight at the same time that they are hailed as the remedy to urban economic decline. Their operations direct the fiscal futures of their host cities to underwriting medical tourism and franchising overseas facilities and hospitality services. As such, it is imperative to weigh the spatially and fiscally predatory operations and effects of Eds and Meds development projects. Even policies such as health-fields, which hold the promise of local land governance and health access, also tether waste management and environmental benefits to the efficient turnover of land for property value growth, which can lead to land use deracination and community displacement on top of inadequate cleanups that are obscured from public oversight.

Projects that rely on determinations of blight not only potentially exacerbate the problems they claim to remedy and/or harm neighborhoods; such a domestic colonialism also anchors transnational speculative development projects and medical investment frontiers that further intensify global health stratification. Clearly a transnational approach is needed to address U.S. health inequities as well as the territorial, socioenvironmental organization of medical services and clinical practices. From a methodological stance, this involves positioning the typically national framework of public health within the political economy of global health and various legacies of empire and domination; it also involves considering the relations of health stratification across scales, be they local, regional, national, or global. The approach requires demythologizing the educational nonprofit mission of U.S. academic hospitals and confronting the violent tautologies of hospital land use that maintain the property frontier and perpetuate vast asymmetries. Because North American racial formations are connected to global racial projects, land policies and development practices of American hospitals succeed in accumulating capital: they drain public resources from national health systems to advance global medical markets while providing nominal emergency care within the United States' minimal social safety net. This entrenches a global color line connecting domestic blight to medical tourism, tethering medical brownfields to global medical entrepôts. While claiming that benefits will trickle down, medical joint ventures extend the domestically extractive processes of U.S. hospitals transnationally, further dividing the medical haves from the have-nots in terms of the structural violence of interrelated forms of harm to embodied health. Yet the moralizing discourse of medical progress and educational mission thwarts consideration of the active role of the U.S. health care system in despoiling the conditions necessary for the right to health.

What would the U.S. health system look like if it were based on "nonkilling" rather than the wasting and devaluation of certain groups?[9] How might Western medicine's ethical imperative to do no harm better address the forms of health colonialism I have examined here? How might consideration of the role of health care in making and maintaining health inequities be tied to the pursuit of their unmaking through policy and practice?[10] First, rethinking

9. James Tyner and Joshua N. Inwood, "Introduction to Nonkilling Geographies: Opening New Spaces," in *Nonkilling Geography*, edited by James Tyner and Joshua N. Inwood (Honolulu: Center for Global Nonkilling, 2011), 11–18.

10. Shiloh Krupar and Amina Sadural, "Covid 'Death Pits': U.S. Nursing Homes, Racial Capitalism, and the Urgency of Antiracist

liberal definitions of harm offers an important starting point, one that shifts focus from individual responsibility to broader social-structural relationships. Further, instead of diagnosing harm as the unfortunate failure or disruption of the universal benefits of U.S. medicine, we might instead heed the way harm maintains the health system and how medical institutions have been complicit in histori-cal and ongoing social and ecological violence. This speculative turn would highlight the harmful promises that underpin global health's claims to universalism. Extending the supposedly universal benefits of global health to more people does not uproot what Kim TallBear calls the "deadly hierarchies of life" that are the existing system's foundation.[11] Within the political economy of health and empire, the fulfillment of modern promises continues to rely on and reproduce divisions of humanity—positioned outside of the realm of ethical obligation and political rights—that are exploitable for the sake of "progress."[12] We see this in the stark accounts of social determinants of health that frequently and falsely attribute violence to the people who are subjected to it, the result of being impoverished, displaced, or disposed by intersecting settler-colonial racial-capitalist frontiers and administrative systems of rule.[13]

Second, in order to unlearn violent ideologies, desires, and infra-structures and relearn different ways of being together in the world, inquiries about health and care should also strive to decenter liberal ideas about public goods, civic benefits, and public lands and use.[14] Public health draws on notions of the public good to make polit-ical and ethical demands; indeed, advocates contend that health is a public good. Yet efforts to reclaim advantages and assurances against privatization—to resist neoliberal accumulation premised

---

Eldercare," *Environment and Planning C: Politics and Space* 40, no. 5 (2022), https://doi.org/10.1177/23996544211057677.

11. Kim TallBear, "Caretaking Relations, Not American Dreaming," *Kalfou* 6, no. 1 (2019): 26; Stein, "Confronting," 90.

12. Stein, "What Can Decolonial," 395.

13. Stein, "Confronting," 82.

14. Stein, "What Can Decolonial," 397.

on the privatization of what was once deemed public—all too often engage in "colonial unknowing" by failing to address the ongoing violence of what is considered civics, public use, the commons, or blight improvement. Following Stein, "it is necessary to ask not only who is the 'public,' and who has the power to decide what is 'good,' but also, who bears the costs of achieving this 'good'?"[15] Constantly referring to public health or global health as doing good similarly forecloses conversations about structural violence related to the political economy of philanthrocapitalism and the colonizing logic of a global medical commons defined by Western biomedicine.[16] It is challenging and controversial to suspend default assumptions about medical institutions doing good, especially in the face of teleological reverence for technological progress and medical advancements in saving lives. I have sought to disrupt liberal nostalgia for public goods and civic moralism by denaturalizing accumulation, white property, and divisions of humanity that undergird U.S. health care regardless of public/private or profit/nonprofit distinctions.

Third, reconceiving global health as an ongoing commitment and process means questioning liberalism's "implicit horizons of justice, hope, futurity, and change."[17] Challenging U.S. health care entails reckoning with the Western biomedical model and cultivating better understandings and practices of health without resorting to heroic liberal subjects and sacrifice. The liberal tradition entails social relations of property that desocialize medicine and that partition the body from ecology and embodied health from the environment and politics. The Western division between medical ethics and broader socioenvironmental ethics means that U.S. biomedicine and the health care system do not address their institutional effects as situated practices that actively influence health conditions. The disavowal of their role in urban political ecologies and property frontiers can justify confiscation of land, devaluation of labor, and

15. Stein, "Confronting," 89.
16. Stein, "What Can Decolonial," 406.
17. Daffé, Guillaume, and Ivers, "Anti-racism," 559; Stein, "What Can Decolonial," 388.

uneven distribution of disease and illness, even as they conduct the work of saving lives and supporting wellness. Thus, it is imperative to elevate the ideal of "do no harm" beyond the notion of helping others. "Do no harm" must prioritize eliminating oppressive systems; rediscover roots in social medicine and collective health; and engage in forms of solidarity committed to social change as the only potentially therapeutic approach to many health problems, whether human, ecological, or planetary.[18] Rather than reducing health services to hospitals or aid organizations, we would instead consider public health everywhere, thus galvanizing specific geographies of justice-oriented decolonial, ecological, and reparative efforts within and beyond biomedicine.[19]

While the adoption of antiracism as an explicit value in global health has led to important introspections on altruistic motivations, charity, aid, and wanting to do good, this work too easily accepts the status quo of deep economic injustices that have created power and resource imbalances.[20] A fourth implication of this book is that any platform for raising global antiracist priorities in health policy—and growing health systems grounded in solidarity—must address the land practices of medical institutions and their role in intensifying the global color line within the context of medical investment frontiers that remain dependent on capitalist imperatives. Without this critical interrogation, this nonredistributive antiracism can serve as ideological cover for the expansion of U.S. medical brownfield frontiers at home and abroad, thus disguising humanitarian imperialism with developmentalist rhetoric and aesthetics, discrediting public institutions, subjugating care workers to further financial-

18. Waitzkin and Jasso-Aguilar, "Empire, Health, and Health Care," 274; Tim Lang, "Public Health and Colonialism: A New or Old Problem?" *Journal of Epidemiology and Community Health* 55 (2001): 162.

19. Sara Elisa Fischer, Poorvaprabha Patil, Chris Zielinski, et al., "Is It About the 'Where' or the 'How'? Comment on *Defining Global Health as Public Health Somewhere Else*," *BMJ Global Health* 5 (2020), https://doi.org/10.1136/bmjgh-2020-002567.

20. Daffé, Guillaume, and Ivers, "Anti-racism," 558.

administrative logics of extraction, and undermining the common sense of universal health coverage.[21]

As key players in urban economies, hospitals, such as the non-profits I target for criticism, are a crucial sector within struggles for liberation and the politics of land. As Frantz Fanon has made clear, the most essential value of a colonized people is "first and foremost the land" because it "will bring them bread and, above all, dignity."[22] Using Fanon as an ecocritical muse, Stephanie Clare continues: "Dignity is not about 'embodying a set of values.' It has 'nothing to do with human dignity.' . . . The dignity of land . . . is the dignity of not being 'arrested, beaten, and starved with impunity.'"[23] It is the dignity of simply living and transforming land and liveli-hood, of refusing to constitute an "inert panorama" or backdrop within which colonizers live.[24] For Fanon, "life" is the quality of being directed toward the future, activated by relations with land that support "breathing and bread."[25] Reorienting hospitals toward "breathing and bread" could entail things like shared governance with their surrounding communities; support for public low-cost medical education; divestment from the financial category of blight as the rationale for land seizure and tax-increment financing; and growing health care facilities as land rematriation trusts, limited equity cooperatives, and other ways of liberating territory to support "the life-sustaining and life-giving work of caring for the land and

21. Jodi Melamed, *Represent and Destroy: Rationalizing Violence in the New Racial Capitalism* (Minneapolis: University of Minnesota Press, 2011), 4; Stein, "Confronting," 87; Neil Singh, "Medicine and Public Health at the End of Empire," *Critical Public Health* 25, no. 4 (2015): 507.

22. Frantz Fanon, *The Wretched of the Earth*, translated by Constance Farrington (New York: Grove, 1963), 44.

23. Stephanie Clare, "Geopower: The Politics of Life and Land in Frantz Fanon's Writing," *Diacritics* 41, no. 4 (2013): 69.

24. Clare, "Geopower," 71; Frantz Fanon, *Toward the African Revolution*, translated by Haakon Chevalier (New York: Monthly Review Press, 1967), 125.

25. Clare, "Geopower," 63, 69.

caring for each other."[26] Given the global justice dimensions of U.S. policy on health care, debt cancellation offers another crucial way to prioritize solidarity over profitability and everyday collective forms of health over empire, to "free up critical public fiscal space for countries to invest in their health and care infrastructure systems," especially for countries hard hit by Covid and without critical resources to support health care during the pandemic.[27] Policy attentive to the relations between climate change and the racialized, gendered transnational stratification of care labor could also strive to eradicate the occupational segregation that places women of color and other vulnerable migrant care workers internationally in such underpaid and devalued essential work, and implement pathways to citizenship. In cases where land is not explicitly the goal, strategies to subvert the practices and rationalities that reduce people to "human debris"—what Sylvia Wynter characterizes as the predicating of "liberal man" on demarcations of human difference—can catalyze spatial reorganizations of colonial geographies.[28] As diverse anticolonial projects and positionalities are well aware, securing more control over the social and political mechanisms that organize human relationships, from political groups to education to care labor, involves rearranging race, property, land, waste, and/or space. My obligation to that work has been to arrange a critical geography of the property frontiers, civic moralism, and transnational development aesthetics of U.S. hospitals, and to invigorate abolition of the mounting global color line of medical apartheid by delineating medical brownfields as the base map of health colonialism.

26. Palladino and Gunn-Wright, "Care and Climate," 5. Huey P. Newton's concept of "liberated territory" is discussed in Safransky, "Rethinking Land Struggle," 1096.

27. Palladino and Gunn-Wright, "Care and Climate," 24.

28. Hannah Arendt, *Origins of Totalitarianism,* 3rd ed. (New York: Harvest, 1994), 150; Sylvia Wynter, "How We Mistook the Map for the Territory, and Reimprisoned Ourselves in Our Unbearable Wrongness of Being, of Desêstre: Black Studies Toward the Human Project," *A Companion to African-American Studies,* edited by Lewis R. Gordon and Jane Anna Gordon (Blackwell, 2006), 107–18.

(Continued from page iii)

Forerunners: Ideas First

Steve Mentz
Break Up the Anthropocene

John Protevi
Edges of the State

Matthew J. Wolf-Meyer
Theory for the World to Come: Speculative Fiction and Apocalyptic Anthropology

Nicholas Tampio
Learning versus the Common Core

Kathryn Yusoff
A Billion Black Anthropocenes or None

Kenneth J. Saltman
The Swindle of Innovative Educational Finance

Ginger Nolan
The Neocolonialism of the Global Village

Joanna Zylinska
The End of Man: A Feminist Counterapocalypse

Robert Rosenberger
Callous Objects: Designs against the Homeless

William E. Connolly
Aspirational Fascism: The Struggle for Multifaceted Democracy under Trumpism

Chuck Rybak
UW Struggle: When a State Attacks Its University

Clare Birchall
Shareveillance: The Dangers of Openly Sharing and Covertly Collecting Data

la paperson
A Third University Is Possible

Kelly Oliver
Carceral Humanitarianism: Logics of Refugee Detention

P. David Marshall
The Celebrity Persona Pandemic

Davide Panagia
Ten Theses for an Aesthetics of Politics

Shiloh Krupar is distinguished associate professor in the culture and politics program at Georgetown University. She is author of *Hot Spotter's Report: Military Fables of Toxic Waste* (Minnesota, 2013), and coauthor of *Deadly Biocultures: The Ethics of Life-Making* (Minnesota, 2019).

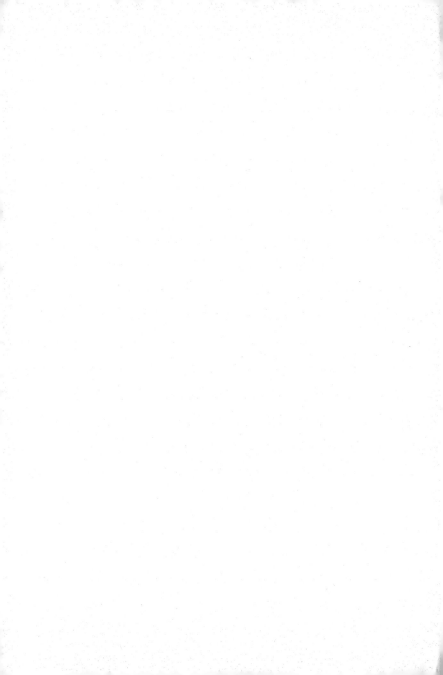